Scientists Must Speak

D0068692

Scientists Must Speak

Bringing presentations to life

D. Eric Walters
Associate Professor of Biochemistry and
Molecular Biology
The Chicago Medical School

Gale Climenson Walters
Manager, Food Technology
COE Nutritionals
Tetra Pak International

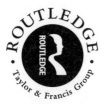

London and New York

First published 2002
by Routledge
11 New Fetter Lane, London EC4P 4EE

Simultaneously published in the USA and Canada
by Routledge
29 West 35th Street, New York, NY 10001

Routledge is an imprint of the Taylor & Francis Group

© 2002 Taylor & Francis

Typeset in Sabon and Gill by BC Typesetting, Bristol
Printed and bound in Great Britain by
TJ International Ltd, Padstow, Cornwall

All rights reserved. No part of this book may be reprinted or
utilised in any form or by any electronic, mechanical,
or other means, now known or hereafter invented, including
photocopying and recording, or in any information storage
or retrieval system, without permission in writing from
the publishers.

British Library Cataloguing in Publication Data
A catalogue record for this book is available from the British Library

Library of Congress Cataloging in Publication Data
A catalog record for this book has been requested

ISBN 0–415–28028–1

Contents

PART III
Special situations 103

Preface

Most scientists and technical workers find their work fascinating and exciting. If you engage such a person in a one-on-one conversation you can often get a strong sense of this excitement. Yet in formal speaking situations the enthusiasm is often suppressed in favor of a deadly serious recitation of dry facts. Some people are simply not trained to handle public speaking situations. Others fear that too much enthusiasm might call their scientific objectivity into question. This book aims to help you present your technical information in clear, credible language and to convey the passion you feel for your subject.

We have been fortunate in recent years to learn from the students who have enthusiastically participated in our "Technical Presentations" course. They offered much constructive feedback on draft versions of this book. In particular, we wish to thank Dr Leyla Akman, Dr Roopa Bhat, Dr Jonathan Boomer, Dr Lihong D'Angelo, Dr Zhihong Deng, Yan Dong, Amy Dressel, Laura Dvorak, Laura Eriks, Mark Fons, Dr Alison Hinds, Dr Steve Kantor, Yoon Sang Kim, Nandan Lad, Steven Latshaw, Dr Gerald Lee, Qiuping Li, Dr Lana Louie, Chunlong Ma, Dr Art Mandelin, Siu Ng, Dr Tao Nguyen, Dr Evangelos Ntrivalas, Dr Fikret Sahin, Dr Zhilin Song, Dr Christy Stine, David Tampa, Dr Yongjun Tan, Tara Teppen, Dr Reha Toydemir, Houman Vaghefi, Mina Wang, Dr Xiaojun Wang, Huaqiang Wen, Kefang Xie, and Daesong Yim. We would also like to thank Anne Wilson, Dr Howard Kanare, Dr David Jacobs, and Dr Frank Kotsonis for their encouragement in this project, and especially Deb Pauley for her careful reading of the entire manuscript.

Introduction
It begins with attitude!

Why are so many technical presentations so dull? There are several reasons. When you speak on a scientific or technical subject your presentation must be precise. The data, equations, graphs, chemical structures, diagrams, blueprints, or formulas that might be necessary to support your key points must be accurate. The presentation must cover material that a lay audience might consider esoteric. You will have to use words that are not part of everyday conversation. As a professional, you want your listeners to take you seriously. Does this mean that your talk is destined to be boring and lifeless? Absolutely not! Presumably there is a reason why you yourself are interested in the topic to be discussed. Why *did* you choose to study this subject? Why did you work on this project for the last three years? Something about the topic got you interested and excited. The key is for you, the speaker, to convey that excitement to your listeners. *If you can get your listeners to feel the same enthusiasm that you do about your subject, your presentation will come to life!*

Why does it matter?

In your scientific or technical career you probably spend only a small percentage of your time in formal speaking situations. However, these situations can have a tremendous impact on your career. If you speak well, you enhance your credibility. If you communicate clearly, you increase your visibility both within your organization and in the larger professional community. Good presentation skills can show others why your work is important or exciting. And an oral presentation is interactive, providing immediate opportunity for you to clear up questions or misunderstandings about your work. Best of all, you have the opportunity to make your work come to life for the listener. *People will be much more influenced by your 20-minute description of your research than by your 20-page paper on the same subject.*

When do I need these skills?

In addition to the occasional formal presentation you will find *numerous* other situations where speaking skills increase your effectiveness. Do you update your supervisor on your progress at departmental or research group meetings? Do you present in-house seminars or lead journal club discussions? Are you preparing for a thesis defense? Are you involved in teaching or training? It is particularly important to be able to communicate technical work to people who do not have highly technical backgrounds. You may have to gain support for your project from a corporate vice-president or a research foundation, calm customers' fears about the safety of one of your company products, or you may be invited to speak to a junior high school science class.

Many speaking opportunities call upon you to speak about your work informally and without preparation. Do you do technical sales or support work? Do you talk about your work with your colleagues over lunch? Do you ever interview for a new position, either inside or outside of your current organization? Suppose the vice-president of research and development drops by with a visitor and asks you to tell the guest about your project. You must be able to describe concisely what you do and explain why it is important and exciting. You must also quickly assess your listener's level of comprehension and choose the appropriate level of detail. For many people this is an intimidating situation. If you have practiced your speaking skills, you will find such a situation far less stressful. It becomes an opportunity to make a favorable impression, not only on your visitor but on your boss as well.

In all situations, if you are an effective communicator you greatly enhance your professional image. Unfortunately, the converse is true: *an excellent technical professional who cannot communicate ideas may hide his or her talents and fail to be taken seriously.*

How can I improve?

The first step in becoming a better speaker is really simple: you must decide that you *want* to be better. Once you have made this decision you will look at speaking situations in a completely different light. If you sincerely *want* to communicate with your audience your *sincerity* will show, and sincerity alone goes a long way toward getting the audience on your side.

Another change takes place when you consciously decide to become a better speaker. You begin to notice the strengths and weaknesses of other speakers. You pay attention to the techniques that contribute to clear, informative talks. You notice things that detract from good communication. This is a hidden benefit of working on your speaking skills – you will never have to be bored during a speech again! If the topic of the talk is not interesting to you, you can study the speaker's presentation skills. What is being done well? What could be improved? Is the material well organized? Do the visual aids support the message? Has the speaker chosen clear language? You can learn something from *every* speaker you listen to! It's also an excellent opportunity to support the development of other speakers. After a presentation, if you are in a position to have a private conversation with the speaker, praise specific aspects of a presentation that you appreciated. If you can identify what would have helped you enjoy the presentation even more, you may consider offering constructive suggestions as well. For instance, suggesting that a particular slide might have carried more impact if divided into two slides can assist the speaker in reaching the audience. If you are interested in the business and art of making presentations your enthusiasm will be contagious. Communication will improve, and that is desirable for all involved!

It is important to emphasize at the outset of this book that speaking is something you learn by *doing*. Reading this book is just a starting point. Becoming a better speaker is an ongoing process, much like becoming a better golfer or a better piano player. You may never reach perfection, but you can get much better by practicing and by observing others. In fact, "perfection" is a false and misleading goal – the real goal is *progress*. Roger Ailes, who has coached presidents and corporate leaders, observes that the real goal should be to put *yourself* into your presentation – to be "you at your best."

To become "you at your best" from a speaking perspective, you must practice, practice, practice. This means rehearsing your formal presentations, and it means looking for opportunities to speak. If you are having difficulty finding opportunities to practice speaking, find a local chapter of Toastmasters International (www.toastmasters.org). Toastmasters Clubs bring together people from many different professions with the goal of helping people improve their speaking skills in a supportive atmosphere. Members practice giving speeches, and they practice giving constructive evaluations of their fellow members' speeches. The Toastmasters Club is a terrific forum for beginners and experts to build their speaking skills.

What will this book do for me?

This book resulted from our experiences with scientific presentation situations in corporate and academic settings. We have had the good fortune to learn from many excellent teachers and speakers. We have also learned a great deal in recent years from working with students in our course, "The Art of Scientific Presentation." We videotape our student presentations on the first day of class and on the final day, then sit with each student to compare the "before" and "after" presentations. There is always tremendous progress in the clarity and organization of each talk. More importantly, there is an obvious change in the confidence of each speaker. Students who are not native English speakers learn to overcome language barriers and communicate their points clearly. This book will show you how to prepare for your presentation and improve your speaking style. It will help you to prepare good visual aids and use them effectively. It will describe ways to overcome language barriers and deal with stressful situations such as question-and-answer sessions. It will prepare you to go out and speak and gain speaking *experience*.

With experience comes confidence and positive comments from people who have been listening to you. You may even find that you are invited out to speak more often, or that people show enthusiasm when they hear that you are to be the speaker at an event. Soon you will find yourself looking forward to speaking opportunities. You may still experience nervousness, but it will feel more like excitement and anticipation than dread. It will be especially gratifying to find that when you work hard to share what you know with an audience and help them feel your excitement about the subject, they will enthusiastically share what they know with you. *Your speaking situations will trigger new discussions, new insights, new collaborations, and new friendships. You will have become a communicator!*

Some key messages from the introduction

- *Your peers will be much more influenced by your 20-minute description of your research than by your 20-page paper on the same subject.*
- *An excellent technical professional who cannot communicate ideas may obscure his or her talents and fail to be taken seriously.*
- *Your speaking situations will trigger new discussions, new insights, new collaborations, and new friendships. You will become a communicator!*

Part I

Preparation

This section of the book deals with the preparation you do *before* a presentation. These preparation steps are important in making your presentation clear, but they have another positive result. They direct your energies away from worrying about yourself and in the direction of giving something useful to the audience. Focusing your attention *outward* is one of the secrets of dealing with "stage fright" and of putting the audience on your side.

Start your preparation early. Once you start organizing your talk, you will find out that there are things you need to research. When you start practicing your presentation, you may discover that some of your visual aids need to be revised. You may find that your talk is too long or too short, and it needs to be substantially modified. If you wait until the last minute, your audience will sense your lack of preparation and may feel that you were not sincerely interested in them.

This section contains four chapters. We have chosen the order of these four chapters deliberately. Speakers are often tempted to start with one or more graphs or pictures showing the key results, and then they build a talk around those pictures. We believe it is most important to go through the *targeting* process first (Chapter 1). Find out about your audience and decide what you want to tell them. Targeting leads you to your key message, which makes the *organization* process (Chapter 2) very easy to do. Third, you can decide what, if any, *visual aids* should be prepared to illustrate and support your talk (Chapter 3). The final step, *practice* (Chapter 4), will help you refine your message and will prepare you for your presentation.

Chapter 1

Target your talk

If you decide to build a house and you make an appointment to talk with a builder, does the builder come to the first meeting with truck-loads of lumber, concrete, carpet, and roofing? Of course not! First the builder has to find out what kind of house you want. Where will it be built? Will it be a ranch, a split-level, a two-story? How many bedrooms, bathrooms, closets? Brick exterior or aluminum siding? Decisions have to be made, and there has to be a plan. You need to know what the *target* is. Similarly, if you are planning to give a talk you have to determine some things beforehand. Who are you talking to? What are they expecting from you? What do you want the outcome to be? In short, what is your target? In this chapter, we look at the following questions:

1   Who is your audience? What do they want from this presentation?
2   What do you want to accomplish? What is your intended take-home message?
3   How can you meet your listeners' needs *and* accomplish your goals?

Once these questions have been answered your talk will be much easier to prepare. You will know what your target is, and your presentation will become more than simply a recitation of facts.

Who is your audience?

The first focus should be on your audience. If you can understand who they are and what they need, it will be much easier for you to communicate effectively with them.

What brings them together?

What brings these people together in this place at this time? What common interests do they have? Are they all members of the same department or organization? Are they interested in a product or an idea you are promoting? Are they evaluating you as a potential employee or co-worker? Are they hoping to learn something specific from you? Answering these questions will help you to understand their needs and expectations.

What is the occasion for this presentation? A small weekly group meeting may lend itself to a very informal style. Your audience may expect to hear your recent results, and they may want to participate in discussion of that work. Such a talk may be less structured and more interactive. On the other end of the spectrum, your Nobel Prize acceptance speech may be quite a formal lecture. The nature of the event will have a bearing on the style you employ, and on the expectations that your audience brings to your talk.

If the audience happens to be your everyday co-workers, or a classroom full of students who have met some specific prerequisites, it may not be too difficult to assess your listeners properly. But other situations may not be so clear-cut. In a job interview situation, you may be asked in advance to prepare a formal talk about your previous work, or you may be asked on the spur of the moment to give a 20-minute discussion of your current project; you will almost certainly have occasion to talk one-on-one about your technical topic. On other occasions you may be invited to speak to a group whose interests are quite different from yours. An example would be the computational chemist who was asked to speak at a conference on applied mathematics – he had always considered himself to be "just a chemist." It had not occurred to him prior to that moment that he was an expert in applied mathematics! For each situation you should assess who your audience is before you start talking.

Ask questions about the audience in advance

How do we get a good understanding of who the audience will be? The answer is to *ask*. Ask the person who arranged the event. Ask the person who invited you to participate. Ask people who will be in the audience, ask people who have spoken to this group previously, ask anyone and everyone who may have any information at all about your audience. Just as you might ask for a second opinion before having major surgery, you should ask more than one person about your audience. You will get a broader perspective and will have a much clearer picture of who will be listening.

Ask very specific questions. When you ask who will be in the audience you may get a non-specific answer such as "Oh, just the engineers in our department." Ask for names, and ask about their backgrounds. What kinds of engineering are they involved in? What interests do they have besides engineering? You should also ask if there will be non-technical people in the audience. If so, what will be their reasons for coming?

Ask some more questions about your audience. Find out how many people are likely to be present. This will help you in your mental preparation for the event. If you anticipate speaking to ten people and suddenly face a full auditorium, you may feel overwhelmed. Conversely, if you expect a big crowd and only a few people show up you may feel disappointed; you would certainly not want your disappointment to convey the impression you are unhappy about being with those who came.

How technical is this audience?

How much does your audience already know about your topic? Will they have some prior knowledge of your work? Will they be familiar with your competitors' work? Will they have strong opinions on the subject, pro or con? These questions are important in targeting the technical level of your presentation. Too technical, and you lose your audience immediately; too simplistic, and you risk sounding condescending. It would be easy if they all had identical backgrounds, of course. In reality, you will often have some experts and some novices in your audience. The key is quickly to review the basics (without being too simplistic), get everyone to some reasonable level, and then go on from there. It is far more common for scientific and technical speakers to overestimate the audience's familiarity with their subject and to assume everybody knows the basics. This is because we forget how hard we worked to become familiar with our topic. We instinctively fear that others know a lot more than we do. But they've all been working hard to get familiar with their own favorite topics, not yours. It is better to err on the side of starting at a simpler level. Those who are already very familiar with the material will assume you are doing this for the benefit of others who know less than they.

What does the audience want from this presentation?

Now that you have an idea *who* your audience is, it's time to look at what they want from you. What are their expectations? What are their needs? Why are they coming to hear you speak? You may be surprised to learn that they are expecting "a good show!"

According to Carl Sindermann, technical and scientific audiences are basically the same as any theatrical or sports audience. They have a fundamental interest in the event at hand, they often have made financial, time and other sacrifices to be present, and they expect a professional performance. They could get the facts of your subject more quickly and accurately by reading your publications. They are coming because they want to feel your experience, to know something about *you*, and to hear your perspective on the subject. In addition, they may wish to ask questions to clarify their understanding of your subject.

What are the *specific* expectations of your audience? A meeting with the manager of the Engineering Department could require preparation of drawings and succinct reasons or arguments for your plan. On the same project, the president of the company may only want to see the budget proposal for the installation of the machinery depicted in the drawings, and an overview of the general differences between the new machinery and what is being replaced. This brings up another good detail to investigate. Does the audience expect graphs or other special visual aids, or a product demonstration? Imagine the disappointment of the marketing group if they expect that you are bringing a sample of your latest food ingredient breakthrough, and you bring the formula on a piece of paper. Similarly, if full-color graphs of weekly progress are customarily used at the Monday meetings but you throw together impromptu freehand drawings on a transparency, your presentation may appear unprofessional. If you are convinced that a departure from the usual style will be effective you may need to find a clever way to introduce your listeners to the new way of presenting information.

And what is your status likely to be at the presentation? The speaker is not always the honored guest at a speaking occasion. There are times when the speaker is expected to sell an idea, a project, or a product. You might be required to defend a technical or scientific opinion. Or you might be asked to provide informed commentary on a controversial topic. Special thought and preparation should be given to the types of questions that may be asked when the audience is likely to be uninformed, skeptical, angry, or emotional in some other way.

What do you want to accomplish?

Now it is time to focus on the second question: what do *you* hope will happen as a result of your talk? Identify your objectives and be able to summarize your message in a single, clear sentence. In your role as speaker you have both the opportunity and the responsibility to determine what the take-home message is. Many technical speakers succumb to the temptation to tell everything they know about a subject. The key points become buried under a mountain of detailed descriptions of experimental procedures. The speaker tries to present as much information as possible, hoping the listeners will select what they want from it. This cafeteria-style approach usually produces one of the following results:

- *Annoyance:* what is the point of this talk?
- *Bewilderment:* what is the point of this talk?
- *Boredom:* what is the point of this talk?

Certainly, circumstances or occasion may put constraints on what that message is to be. If you have only 20 minutes to talk about peptide antibiotics you can't afford to spend very much time reviewing the history of antibiotic discovery. Listeners cannot possibly come away from your 20-minute talk knowing everything about your topic in as much detail as you do! What is the central thing you want them to remember an hour, a day, or a month after your talk? What is your *take-home message*? What do you want your listeners to know, think, feel, believe, or do as a result of your talk?

This is a particular problem for the young scientist preparing a presentation for a job interview. You want to show how much work you did in your research project! But it is much more impressive to give a clear presentation of one aspect of your work. You can allude to other parts of the project in your introduction, and discuss the rest of your work at other points in the interview process. They'll *really* be impressed when they find out you did more work than you could possibly cover in a 40-minute talk.

Start preparing your presentation by going to the end – what do you want your listener to come away with? Whether the goal of your talk is to sell, teach, train, inform, persuade, or entertain, it should be possible to summarize your take-home message in a *single simple sentence*. Practice identifying the key sentence for your presentations and for other lectures you listen to. If you are selling a line of laboratory equipment, your message may be "The Cornell line of moisture analyzers will provide increased accuracy at a lower cost-per-sample and in one-fourth the time." In a job interview presentation, your message might be "I am a creative, productive, and persistent experimentalist." Of course, you wouldn't use that as the title of your talk – that would be too obvious. But if that is the message you really wish to convey, you can describe your research on earthworm socialization in ways which show just how creative, productive, and persistent you were in carrying out that work. The presentation that is built around a well-chosen message and is strongly supported by a few significant facts will benefit both speaker and listener. Once you have a succinct key message, the rest of your task of preparing a presentation becomes much easier, as we will see in Chapter 2.

Learn from the experts

Presidential debates and other political speeches can teach us a great deal about preparing for our presentations. In the typical debate or press conference it appears that the speaker is able to talk extemporaneously in response to every question! It's not really a miracle, though. In reality, the speaker has anticipated most of the *topics* which are likely to be raised, rather than worrying about all possible questions on all possible topics. For each topic, the speaker has committed to memory a *specific message* that can be summarized in one sentence. That message could be something very precise, such as "I am asking the Congress to immediately pass Bill 963, imposing $1 million fines for toxic waste dumping." Or it could be something as content-light as "My party continues to stand for traditional values." It matters not – whatever the question asked, the speaker will be able to construct an answer around the key message which has been worked out in advance. The speaker will also probably conclude the question period with the one-sentence thought he or she wants the listeners to remember. These "key messages" become the basis for the ubiquitous "soundbites" which appear on the television news programs. If interviewers feel that they are not getting a real answer and they persist in asking questions about this topic, the speaker simply uses the opportunity to repeat and reinforce the key message. Nothing stands in the way of delivering the key message!

We could look at this as cynical manipulation of the media. But these speakers know that listeners will not remember long passages of speech. Expect instead that listeners will remember a key sentence or idea. Effective speakers have worked to identify the goal of the speaking occasion, to put a key idea into a concise and memorable form, to build a talk around it, and to highlight and reinforce that idea throughout the talk. Take the time to identify the key message you want your listeners to go home with. Your presentation will be much more focused and you will be better prepared to answer questions in a way that keeps you in control of the presentation opportunity.

How can you meet your listeners' needs *and* accomplish your goals?

Now we have to look at targeting the presentation in such a way that both you and your listeners will be pleased with the results. With a little effort you can usually find a way to make the outcome quite satisfying for everyone involved. The recipe for any successful presentation will need to include several ingredients.

A brief, dynamic introduction to your presentation

Every popular song has a "hook" – a musical phrase which sticks in your mind. The introductory sentences of your talk also need some sort of a "hook" to capture your listeners' attention right from the start. There are many ways to do this. Introduce your talk with a compelling story or a surprising statistic; use an eye-catching and unusual picture to introduce your topic; tell them about the important question or problem that you will be discussing. Then provide a concise summary of the background needed to put your message into a context that is meaningful for your listeners.

Your audience will be lost throughout your whole presentation if they don't find out very quickly what the point of the talk is. Remember the "key message" we discussed earlier in this chapter? Share it with your listeners early in your presentation. The audience appreciates being led quickly and easily to the key message. They are most receptive when they are not wondering what is going on and they can spend their energy focusing on what you are telling them. After the main point becomes clear, the listeners will know how to process all of the supporting information you provide in the body of your talk.

You, the speaker, are also helped by having a clear key message expressed right at the beginning of your talk. Knowing your message adds to your confidence, and it becomes clear to everyone that you know what you want to accomplish. The result is that you have a much better chance of helping the audience to see your point.

Your regard for the audience

The audience might be at a higher energy level at 8 a.m. than they are after a big lunch break or after listening to five other speeches. Be sensitive to their needs, and be energetic for them. Body language can help – large, exuberant gestures convey your energy and your enthusiasm for the topic. Involve your listeners by asking a question or two. Watch for cues that the audience may need a pause in your presentation to grasp a concept or to ask a question. In lengthy presentations (over an hour), watch for indications that the audience needs a rest break or a change of pace. For a very long presentation (two hours or more), it may be appropriate to take a ten-minute break; in other cases it may be sufficient simply to stop talking and take a few questions.

Your obvious enthusiasm for the topic

You have spent the last ten years of your career investigating the genetic modification of algae. Help the audience feel your excitement for all your dedicated work! If the speaker can't get excited about the topic, how can he expect the listeners to find it interesting? Projecting excitement is a particularly difficult task for many technically trained speakers; we sometimes think we have to be very reserved if we are to be taken seriously. Perhaps this is because we associate an enthusiastic presentation with commercial advertising, which we know is not at all scientific! But pay attention to those technical people whom you consider to be "good speakers." Most of the time, what makes them effective is that they let the audience see just how excited they are about their favorite topic. It may take a lot of effort for you to let your enthusiasm show. If showing enthusiasm is difficult for you, try these exercises. First, in an empty classroom or conference room, with an imaginary audience, say "I really like this subject!" Smile, laugh out loud, and, if necessary, shout it out! Next, when you practice your talk, start with the sentence "I really like working on (or talking about) this topic because . . ." (fill in why you like your topic). When you take the time to consider why you chose this topic, and then share that reason with your listeners, you begin to let them see what's so great about it, and your enthusiasm adds life to your presentation.

It really is critical for you to feel enthusiasm about your topic. If you don't feel it, your audience will sense this and your presentation will suffer. Find *something* exciting about your topic. At the very least, be glad for the opportunity to share what you know with this particular group of people. Put some zip into your arrow as you aim it toward the target. You want your message to pierce the bull's-eye, not just bump up against it and fall to the ground.

Emphasis on the significant conclusions

Although your original work might have been published as an authoritative 600-page book, your mission in an oral presentation is to help the audience remember vividly a few key results or conclusions. No oral presentation will ever provide you with enough time to tell everything you know, so you have to be selective. Narrow the scope of your presentation; select one or two experiments and describe them clearly rather than racing through 15 different procedures. Since you are with the audience in person, you can clear up questions and misunderstandings about the topic if this is required. Details are important when *publishing* technical work, but they are deadly boring in an oral presentation. This is true even in a classroom lecture. The lecturer should put the subject into perspective, tell which details are important, explain why they are important, and indicate where the details can be found. It would be pointless for the lecturer to read from the textbook or to recite a table of data! When you highlight the important points, you make your subject come to life for the audience. Present the key results in an easily understood style, and leave the details to a written format.

Words that reach every person in the audience

One of the most difficult aspects of technical presentation is to be sure you are neither too technical nor too simplistic. You want to reach each person on his or her own level of understanding. If you are sure that all members of the audience have the same level of knowledge you can safely use technical terminology. In general, however, strictly limit your use of acronyms and jargon. Be sure to explain any abbreviations or terms you do use, unless you are positive everyone is familiar with them. If you plan to refer to "recent results from Tony Dean's lab," you should ask yourself whether *everyone* in the audience will know who and what you mean, or whether you need to elaborate a little on what those results are.

Once we become familiar with a subject we forget how hard we worked to pick up the basics. We lose sight of those aspects that may not be quite so familiar to our audience. Some things seem so simple to us in hindsight that we assume everybody must already know them. But most of the time your listeners haven't had the same experiences you have had. Even if they have some familiarity with your subject or your field, they probably do not know the details as thoroughly as you think they do. Thus, it is important to practice your talk in front of people who are less familiar with your subject so that they can bring to your attention questions about abbreviations or jargon such as: "What does FIP stand for?" "What is a Southern Blot?" "What is a Morse potential?" "What is a back-of-the-envelope calculation?" Audiences are rarely homogeneous, so most of the time we have to give at least a quick review of the basics. To you, it is painfully obvious why one should study the substrate specificity of dihydrofolate reductase; most audiences, however, would appreciate a sentence or two in which you explain the significance of this subject.

Minimum details of "techniques"

We usually should not get to the level of detail that we as experts are capable of reaching. Esoteric descriptions of how experiments were designed and executed are generally difficult to follow (and they are also frequently very dull!). An exception would be if the design of the experiment *is* the significant discovery. In that case, salient comparisons to the former way of doing the experiment, or making clear that no suitable methods existed previously, could be made very interesting.

The "minimal details" rule becomes especially important in situations where the audience is largely non-technical. Their lack of a technical background does not entitle you to be condescending, nor to leave them in the dark. Find out what their needs are. Find ways to make your message accessible to them as well. Here are some ideas:

- Connect your topic to some everyday phenomenon. For example, if you are discussing a yeast ATPase enzyme, you could relate it to more familiar functions of yeast – beer fermentation, bread rising – or to the role of ATP in burning up calories.
- Make use of analogy. For example, the voltage-sensitive channels which transport potassium ions across cell membranes cycle through three states: first, there is a resting state in which the channel is closed but is sensitive to a change in voltage; second, when the voltage changes the channel goes to an open state, allowing ions to pass through; third, immediately after opening the channel goes to a closed state in which it is *not* sensitive to voltage change. After a recovery period, the channel is again in the resting (voltage-sensitive) state. These three states can be compared to a standard flush toilet: there is a resting state, in which the flap valve is closed but handle-sensitive; there is an open state, in which the valve is open; and there is a closed recovery state, during which handle-activation cannot produce another flush. After the tank refills, the toilet is again in the initial resting state.
- As much as possible, describe your work in everyday language. If you and your colleagues work with asynchronous transfer mode every day you may find it convenient to refer to it as "ATM," but that abbreviation may mean nothing (or perhaps something totally different) to your audience.

When we teach technical presentation skills in the classroom we ask our students to do the following exercise. Select a technical topic to speak about for a period of five minutes. First, give a five-minute speech as though you are speaking to other experts in the field. Next, speak for five minutes on the same topic as though you are speaking to a group of other scientists who are not necessarily working in the same area. Finally, talk on this subject for five minutes as though the audience is a high school science club. What happens? Every member of the class notices that the talks become progressively clearer. In many cases, the last presentation is judged to be the best of the three, even for a highly technical audience. This is one of the secrets of giving a memorable technical talk: *Listeners are more impressed by clarity than by technical detail.*

A succinct, clear summary and reiteration of the "take-home message"

The audience needs to know when your presentation is finished so that they can decide whether they understood your message, if the promised points were made, or if you provided enough information. If you finish your presentation by trailing off vaguely, your listeners will feel let down. They may question your desire to communicate and even your credentials for handling the subject. Don't disappoint them. Give them a punchy ending – a concise, positively worded, solid conclusion that summarizes and reinforces your key message.

Allow five to ten minutes of question and answer time

A speaking situation almost always has a time allotment. One of the most effective uses of your presentation time is to allow a few minutes at selected points during your talk to allow the audience to ask questions, so that they can clarify their interpretation of what you have said. The questions, comments, applause and expressions on the faces of the audience will tell you whether the ideas and conclusions you intended were understood and well received. The audience involvement with your presentation is so important that it is better to cut from the body of your talk, if confronted with a situation where your talk is cut short, than to run out of time to discuss your talk with the audience.

Summary

A professional speaking performance requires planning, practice, more practice and the *desire* to communicate. This desire to communicate will allow you to answer these key questions: What does the audience want from this occasion? What do I want the audience to conclude, remember, feel or act upon as a result of my time with them? How can all of these needs be met in one presentation?

The audience will invest time and effort to attend your presentation. They expect a worthwhile, professional occasion. Investigate the needs of the audience in advance. Discover who the audience is, and decide how best to reach them. Focus the audience on one key take-home message, and support that message with a few well-chosen details, examples, or anecdotes. The power of a clear message and easily grasped supporting material will give you, the speaker, confidence, and it will provide the audience with a high level of comfort.

Some key messages from this chapter

- *Targeting your talk helps to make your presentation more than just a recitation of facts.*
- *What is the central thing you want the audience to remember? That key message must be in the introduction, the body and the conclusion of your presentation.*
- *Listeners are more impressed by clarity than by technical detail.*
- *Question and answer time is so important that it is better to cut from the body of your talk than to run out of time to discuss your talk with the audience.*

Exercises

1   A chemist who uses computer modeling in the design of new drugs has, in recent months, been asked to present lectures to several different groups: (1) a group of computational chemists; (2) an applied mathematics conference; (3) a group of biochemists interested in antiviral drugs; (4) a college science club; (5) a junior high school science class. This chemist identified the following very different "key messages," all of which were drawn from the same body of research results: (1) a new method has been developed for constructing practical models of drug receptor sites; (2) simple force-field equations, plus a genetic algorithm, can generate models which are able to predict the bioactivities of new drugs; (3) newly developed computer methods are aiding in the design of new antiviral drugs; (4) computational chemistry has become an important tool in the design of new drugs; (5) computers can help us see how drugs work and can give us ideas about how to make new drugs.

Using *your* favorite technical topic, construct a "key message" sentence for a 40-minute talk to each of the following groups:

(a) Your current co-workers.
(b) A company which is interviewing you for a job.
(c) A science seminar at your local community college.
(d) A science class at the high school from which you graduated.
(e) A group of venture capitalists who are considering commercialization of your work.

Does each message seem appropriate to the needs of your audience? Does each message serve your needs as well?

2   The next time you attend a lecture or seminar, see whether you can discern the speaker's key message. What did the speaker want you to remember? What was most memorable for you? Did the presentation satisfy both your needs and the speaker's goals?

Chapter 2

Organize your presentation

In Chapter 1 we described the process of identifying your key message. This key message provides a centerpiece around which you can build a well-structured talk. In this chapter we look at several methods for *organizing* a talk. Organization helps your talk flow smoothly, and it helps your listeners to more easily comprehend the message you are sending. We will begin by comparing five different ways to structure your presentation. Next we will look at four ways to collect and focus ideas. Finally, we will show you three ways to revise and refine your *good* speech into a *great* speech. You should experiment with these and choose those which suit your style of working and your needs.

Five formulas for structuring the presentation

There are many different "recipes" for structuring the final presentation. The introduction–body–conclusion approach is both common and useful, so we will look at this method first and in more depth. But there are many other formulas which may be used for particular kinds of presentations, and we will describe four of them.

Introduction–body–conclusion formula . . . or, tell, tell, tell

The introduction–body–conclusion formula is so common it almost seems instinctive. It is used frequently because it is logical and it works well. One of the oldest adages of public speaking is "tell them what you're going to tell them, tell them, then tell them what you told them." The introduction tells them what the talk will be about, the body of the talk gives the information with supporting details, and the conclusion summarizes and restates the main message of the talk. By using repetition you reinforce your key message.

The key message should be in the introduction of your talk, the body of the talk should be built around that key message, and the conclusion should serve to reinforce the key message. Later we will add to this time-tested formula the important subject of transitions.

The introduction

The introduction to your talk is your opportunity to grab your audience's attention and take them along with you. You should have the first sentence or two clearly in mind to make sure you get off to a good start. And those first two sentences should get right to the point, so that listeners are immediately interested in your talk. One effective way to draw your audience in right away is to state your topic as a question – the question which your research set out to answer, or the problem which your new methodology is now able to solve, for instance.

The introduction should, above all else, let the listeners know what your key message is. When you do this you let the audience know that you know where you are going, and this helps to put them at ease.

The introduction should also put your topic into a larger context. Instead of jumping right into a talk about species differences in the enzyme phosphofructokinase, tell why you chose to look at this particular enzyme. If the ultimate goal is to cure an infectious disease, discover regulatory pathways, or show the advantages of your new analytical method, make sure you say so in the clearest possible terms.

Putting your topic into context also means providing enough background information so that everyone will be able to follow the rest of the story. When your project began, someone (maybe you!) knew the reason why. Since that time you have become engrossed in the day-to-day details of making sure that reagents are pure enough, or that the analytical method is reproducible enough, or that the algorithm is robust enough. You have come to know the smallest details, but now it is time to step back (perhaps quite far back) and once again see the big picture so that you can help your audience to see the context into which your talk fits.

Chapter 1 described the process of making sure you do this at the appropriate level for your audience.

Be prepared, too, to give some introductory information about yourself, in case you were not given a proper introduction before your talk. People need to know that you are a credible source of information. It's not necessary to recite your entire educational and work history, but it may be appropriate to say, for example, "I've been working on the problem of food additive stability for the last 16 years." There are many ways to incorporate information about yourself into the introduction. You could mention the name of a mentor who first introduced you to the topic, or describe an early research problem which led you to your current field of study. Your audience is looking for more than just a list of facts – they want to know something about you, and they want to hear *your story*. Don't be reluctant to tell it.

The body

The main part of your talk should usually take the largest portion of the allotted time, and it should tell a story about the purpose of your work and the people involved. Experimental results (positive and negative) can illustrate the story, they can support the story, but they are *not* "the story." A talk which is just a sequential catalog of experimental results is about as exciting as reading a dictionary. Explain *what* experiments you did, *why* you chose them, and *what* you learned from the results. If you are talking about a theory, make it concrete by talking about a practical implication. If you are talking about an experimental result, talk about a practical application of that result. Having the story anchored with real examples and something practical will make it much more real for the audience – they will be able to relate more easily to what you say.

The most memorable presentations talk about what happened to the *people* involved in the story you are telling. For example, several gelling agents were discovered accidentally when the discoverer tried unsuccessfully to wash them down the drain, creating laboratory floods. Inject some humanity into your subject, and your listeners will find it much easier to relate to what you are telling them.

Humor is another way to enliven your presentation. But be sure the humor is (a) funny, (b) relevant, and (c) not offensive. Remember, the listeners are your partners, and it isn't a good idea to offend or alienate your partners. If you must make fun of someone it is safest to make fun of yourself. If you have the slightest question about whether your humor will offend, leave it out.

There should be a logical progression to the story. But, if you are describing the results of your research, resist the urge to make it sound as though you knew from the first day exactly what to do and in what order. If research were so predictable it would be boring. Talk about the way your thinking changed as the project went on, talk about the unexpected results, talk about your setbacks and how you overcame them. Don't be afraid to talk about the still-unresolved questions – your listeners will often give you thought-provoking comments and suggestions which will help you with further development of your work. Besides, if you try to gloss over those parts, some listener will raise them for you in the form of pointed questions. It's better for you to let them know that you are aware of the questions which still need to be addressed.

And keep your key message in sight. Make sure that your story directly relates to that message. If you write a paper using a word processor you may run the final copy through the spell-checker. Once you have completed an outline of the body of your talk, run it through your mental "message-checker" – does each part of the talk support your main message in some way? While you are review-ing, check for continuity. Does the story flow smoothly from one point to the next?

How many main supporting points should you have in the body of your talk? To some extent, this depends on your individual story. Three or four seem to be optimal, and seven is about the max-imum that most people can grasp in one sitting. If you have more than that, consider grouping them into a few major categories, each of which is supported by two or three sub-points. Suppose you were to discuss the nine planets of our solar system. One way to group them would be as follows:

1   Inner planets (Mercury, Venus)
2   Rocky planets (Earth, Mars)
3   Gas planets (Jupiter, Saturn, Uranus, Neptune)
4   Small distant planet (Pluto)

Other ways to group them might be in order of their discovery or exploration, or on the basis of their composition. By grouping them, you make the list seem manageable to the listener.

Your topic may naturally lead you to one particular arrangement, or you may have to choose from several. Here are some common ways to arrange the body of your talk:

- Bottom-up (points of evidence, leading to a conclusion)
- Top-down (conclusion first, then the supporting evidence)
- Location order (for example, human body–chest–heart–aorta–aortic valve)
- Time order
- Logical or sequential order

There is not necessarily one "best" way for you to organize the points in your talk. You may be able to construct a successful presentation in several different ways. If you have always looked at your topic in one way, it might be useful for you to try out a new approach.

The conclusion

This is your chance to cement the key message in your listeners' minds. You can recall the question you raised in your introduction and point out how your work answered the question, or in some other way refer back to your introduction. You can summarize your key findings and relate them to your main point. If you want people to do something (buy a product, try your method, fund further research), now is the time to tell them *very specifically* what you want. Conclude by reiterating your main message.

The conclusion is one of the most important components of your talk. We will discuss timing in more detail later, but we must tell you this right now. If you find yourself pressed for time, do *not* cut out any material from your conclusion. Omit or condense some of the body of your talk, and leave your conclusion intact.

The conclusion is not a place to introduce new material. If you bring up a new topic at this stage of your talk, listeners will wonder if they missed something, and they may become distracted or confused.

How do you let the audience know you are through talking? Many speakers end by thanking their audience, but this is usually not appropriate. After all, you have presumably told them something useful, and *they* should be thanking *you*. Other speakers end by acknowledging the contributions of their co-workers and sponsors. It is certainly appropriate to thank those who have aided you in your work, but if you do this after your conclusion your main message is no longer the last thought you leave them with. Consider doing the acknowledgments as you go along, or just before the conclusion, or even at the beginning of your talk.

What, then, is the best way to end a talk, without simply trailing off the last sentence? Craft a final sentence which captures your real message. Make this a clear, strong sentence. Memorize it. Say it with feeling at the end of your talk. Then stop talking. Most speakers fear this part, because they know it will be followed by two eternal seconds of silence. But if you have concluded with a clear, strong final statement and you simply stop talking, your audience will *know* it is time to applaud.

TRANSITIONS

After you have identified the main parts of your talk (introduction, main points, conclusion), give some thought to your transitions. How will you go from the introduction to the first main point? How will you move from one point to the next? And how will you shift from the body of your talk into the conclusion? Your transitions should be smooth, so that the listener can follow your train of thought from one point to the next. But they should not be subtle. The transitions serve several important functions for the listener.

Transitions provide guideposts which let your audience know where they are. Just as road signs provide reassurance to the traveler ("Chicago 250 miles," "Chicago 110 miles," "Chicago 25 miles"), your transitions will let your listeners know that they are making progress through the points of your presentation. It is important to maintain their comfort level so that they are prepared to keep listening. Transitions can also serve to recapture the attention of those whose thoughts may have started to wander. Transitions let people know that something new is coming right up.

Your transition also gives you a chance to summarize one section before going on to the next. This can be particularly useful if your task is to convey some complex information to your listeners. It gives them a moment to assimilate one point before plunging into the next one. You may even want to use this time to answer any questions before going on.

Four other formulas for organizing your final presentation

The introduction–body–conclusion formula is the most commonly used, but it is by no means the only way to put your talk together. Here we summarize four others for you. Much of what we have previously discussed concerning introductions, conclusions, and transitions applies to these methods as well.

Question and answer

Robert Anholt's book on technical presentation is strongly oriented toward research presentations. He advocates using the introduction to pose a question. The body of the talk then consists of the gradual unfolding of the answer to that question. Very often a research question can be broken down into a series of smaller questions. Answering one question frequently leads us to ask another question, and the answer to that one may raise yet more questions, so this method can be used quite effectively when presenting a body of research findings.

The question-and-answer approach can also be used successfully in a classroom setting. For example, a lecture on blood coagulation could be organized around the following series of questions:

- When you cut or damage your skin, why do you not bleed to death?
- Once the blood starts to coagulate, why doesn't the entire blood supply turn into one huge clot?
- After a blood clot forms, how do you get rid of it?
- What causes the hemophilias (coagulation disorders)?
- How, why, and when can coagulation be regulated with medication?

These questions focus attention on the main points of the lecture, and they invite the audience to keep listening in order to find out the answers.

AIDA

AIDA is an acronym for a method advocated by Ralph Smedley, founder of Toastmasters International. It is particularly suited to speeches in which you want to convince an audience to do something specific. Here is the formula:

Attention	Win the audience's attention
Interest	Arouse their interest
Desire	Create a desire
Action	Stimulate action

Let's work through an example. The main message is "Patent protection on new food additives should be extended because of the many years required to obtain regulatory approval."

Attention: "Although aspartame was discovered in 1965, it did not receive final regulatory approval in the United States until 1981."

Interest: "It is in the public interest to develop new food additives which improve the quality, stability, and purity of foods, and it is also important to carry out the lengthy safety testing which regulatory agencies require before a new additive is approved."

Desire: "We want to keep developing new food additives which improve food quality, and we want to maintain the high safety standards we have enjoyed in this country. To encourage manufacturers to keep developing new products, we must extend their patent coverage in line with the amount of time required to obtain regulatory approvals."

Action: "I want you to write to your elected representatives in support of my proposed legislation which would provide the necessary patent protection."

Borden's ho-hum method

Richard C. Borden, a speech professor at New York University, described this formula, which is based on the four stages of an audience's reaction to a speaker:

Ho-hum	The audience is waiting for a reason to pay attention. Give them one!
Why bring that up?	Why is this topic important? What's in it for the listener?
For instance	Give examples, evidence, or tell a story which supports your point.

So what?　　　　　　　　What do you want them to do about it? Be
　　　　　　　　　　　　specific.

Again, let's try this out on a technical topic. This time, the assign-
ment is to persuade a vice-president of marketing to support research
on your new product idea:

Ho-hum: "How would you like a product which looks like sugar,
　　tastes like sugar, can be used in baking applications, and has
　　only one calorie per gram?"
Why bring that up?: "There is currently no product on the market
　　which meets all of these criteria – it would create a whole new
　　category."
For instance: "Consumers are currently confused about non-sugar
　　sweeteners; some taste bad, some aren't stable when heated,
　　none are able to replace sugar directly in recipes."
So what?: "Give us six months time plus the necessary resources
　　to develop this product in the laboratory, including a research
　　scientist, two technicians, and an engineer."

The motivated sequence

The *motivated sequence* is a five-step method described by Monroe
and Ehinger for organizing a persuasive speech. The five steps are as
follows:

- Getting attention
- Showing a need or problem
- Presenting a solution
- Visualizing the results
- Requesting action or approval

As in the AIDA and Ho-hum methods, the first step is to get
the audience's attention, and the last step is to ask for action. The
differences are in the intermediate steps. Here, a problem is presented, followed by a proposed solution. The speaker's preferred
solution to the problem is then "sold" by visualizing what will
happen when the solution is applied. How might we use this
method?

Getting attention: Last year, on average only 23 percent of department members attended departmental seminars given by our own
students.

Showing a need or problem: An informal survey showed that most
of those who do not attend student seminars found them uninfor-
mative and boring.

Presenting a solution: If we provide training in technical presentation skills our students' presentations will become much more
interesting and useful.

Visualizing the results: Imagine what it would be like if, every
Thursday afternoon, you could count on hearing a lucid and
entertaining description of some new scientific discovery.

Requesting action or approval: Let's offer a technical presentation
course as part of our core curriculum. In addition, each new
student will be provided with a copy of *Scientists Must Speak*
by Walters and Walters.

Don't go through the first four steps and then neglect to ask for what
you want.

Collecting, arranging and focusing your ideas

The first step in organizing your presentation is simply to assemble in
one place all of the material you wish to cover. You may need to pull
together notebooks, do some reading or library work, or talk to
others who have some of the information you need. If you have a
few weeks or months to plan your presentation, label a folder
where you can collect articles and jot down ideas relevant to your
topic. Once you start looking for things, you will accumulate quite
a lot of material.

After you have gathered the information you need, you may find it
helpful to collect and arrange your ideas in two distinct stages: a
creative phase followed by a *critical* (editing) phase. In the first
phase, list everything you can think of which might go into your
talk. Don't evaluate whether any topic belongs or not, don't
question where it should go. Just let the ideas flow as freely as you
possibly can – if you start editing at this stage, you will inhibit
your creativity. It may take considerable conscious effort at first to
resist the urge to edit as you go. Make the effort. In just a few
minutes you will find that the ideas begin to come quite rapidly.

Soon you will have more material on the page than you can possibly cover in one talk.

Then comes the time to apply your critical thought processes: evaluate, edit, and arrange the ideas you have amassed. Choose the order in which points will be presented. Decide which ones support your main message and which ones belong in some other presentation. If you succeeded in unleashing your creativity, you may have to do some serious pruning at this stage. Your creative effort and extra material were not wasted, though; the points which remain will all be strong ones.

Finally you will be ready to focus your material. Here are four different ways to do it. (1) If you are preparing a talk on a very familiar subject, you may be able to write an *outline* without much trouble. (2) For material which you have not previously organized, you may find that the *mind-mapping* method is helpful. (3) If you want to achieve a particular result (persuading or selling, for instance), you may find that the *"start at the end"* method is best suited to your needs. (4) And visual thinkers may be most comfortable with the *storyboard* approach. We encourage you to try several different methods and see what works best for you.

Outlining

The outline is one of the most familiar organizational tools. Almost any talk you can imagine could be built on this general outline:

1   *Introduction*
    (a) What the talk is all about
    (b) Necessary background information
2   *Body: telling and supporting the main message*
    (a) First supporting point
    (b) Second supporting point
    (c) Third supporting point (plus as many supporting points as you think you need, but keep in mind that more than seven points is probably too overwhelming to your audience)
3   *Conclusion*
    (a) Summarize the supporting points
    (b) Reiterate the main message

Note that this simple outline has an introduction, a body, and a conclusion. A good rule of thumb is to spend about 5 percent of your allotted speaking time on the introduction and 5 percent on the conclusion. Audiences become very discouraged when, after 30 minutes, the speaker announces the end of the introductory material – how long will this talk go on? If you need to give this much background before your listeners can understand your message, you should ask yourself if you have selected the right message. Perhaps your goal should have been to educate your listeners about all that background material, or perhaps you needed a simpler message. Could some of that "background" material be incorporated into the body of the talk?

Of course an outline that consists of an introduction, a body, and a conclusion is just a starting point which can be modified to fit many different situations. You might wish to use an attention-getting device or story in your introduction before you tell what the talk is about. You might wish to structure the body of your talk in chronological order, or build up from simpler principles to more complex ones, or start with an overview and work through increasing levels of detail. We will examine some of these formulas later in the chapter. But the introduction–body–conclusion approach is very common, and for good reason. Some sort of introduction is needed to draw in your audience – no one wants to come in at the middle of a story. And without a conclusion your presentation will seem unfinished.

Mind-mapping

Tony Buzan pioneered a creativity tool which he calls "mind-mapping." This is a great method for organizing a talk, writing a paper, or planning a project. You begin by writing your central idea in the middle of a sheet of paper. Every time you think of a subject which relates to that idea, draw a branch and write your subject onto it. As you think of sub-points relating to one of your ideas, put them on branches coming off a main idea branch. If two of your branches seem to be closely related, you may wish to draw a dotted line connecting them. Or you may wish to move some small branches from one big branch to another. At this stage, just let the ideas flow freely, and keep adding branches wherever you think they may fit. Let's work through an example.

Suppose our key message is to be "Chemists can give entertaining presentations" (see Figure 2.1). We begin by writing this in the center of the page. How can we support this message? First, many

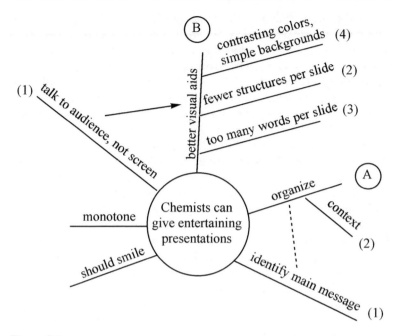

Figure 2.1

chemists need to improve their visual aids, so we draw a branch and label it "better visual aids." We know that one of the worst things chemists may do is to put too many structures on one slide, so we draw a sub-branch and write "fewer structures per slide." That reminds us that chemists, like many other scientists, often have too much text on a slide, so we quickly add a branch which says "too many words per slide." Note that we don't worry about details such as parallel construction ("fewer structures" vs. "too many words") at this point – we are just putting things on paper as rapidly as they come to mind. We remember a recent chemistry seminar we attended and immediately add branches labeled "monotone" and "should smile." Next, we recall that the speaker really needs to identify the main message of the talk, so we put on a branch for that. A branch is added for "talk to audience, not to screen," and then one for "organize." We recall far too many talks where the speaker just jumped right into the middle of a talk without ever telling us why we might be interested in the subject, so we add a sub-branch labeled "context" onto the "organize" branch. Then we realize that "identify the main message" is closely related to organization, so we draw a dotted line connection between those two branches. We may add other points to the "better visual aids" branch as we go along. The process continues until we can't think of anything else which might be relevant. Note that we did not have to think of things in any kind of order. This approach is very freeing – you may find that mind mapping is useful in overcoming writer's block when you are stuck on a writing project.

Now we can begin to edit and evaluate. Which branches are the most important? Which ones ought to be discarded? In our example we may decide that we cannot cover everything in a 15-minute talk, so we will focus on *organization* and *visual aids*. The "monotone" and "smile" branches will be discarded. And the "talk to audience, not to screen" branch can be added to the visual aids section. We can look at the remaining branches and quickly decide what order to put them in, labeling them A–B–C, and we can number the sub-branches 1–2–3. We can combine branches which belong together. From here, it is *very* easy to generate a traditional outline which will easily provide enough material for our short talk, approximately 30 minutes:

1   *Introduction: chemists can give exciting presentations*
2   *Body: how to improve presentations*
   (a) Organize the talk
     • Identify the main message
     • Put the work into context
   (b) Use visual aids effectively
     • Talk to the audience, not the screen
     • Use one or two large structures per slide
     • Use just a few words per slide, using large, clear typeface
     • Use contrasting colors and simple backgrounds
3   *Conclusion: chemists* can *give exciting presentations*

Start at the end and work backwards

Here is an organization method which is especially useful when your goal is to *persuade* your audience or to *sell* a technical idea or product. You already know what you want the conclusion to be: "The trace elements scandium and thorium should be added to municipal water supplies," or "The federal government must support research into extraterrestrial life forms in New Mexico," or "You need to buy the Galaphonic Model 227 audio-spectrum analyzer." Work back from your conclusion. What supporting points must you put in the body of your talk to sustain this conclusion? What questions should you raise (and answer) to lead the audience to the same conclusion you have come to? What kind of introduction do you need to interest your audience in this topic in the first place?

David Peoples describes this method in some detail. He likens it to "setting up the bowling pins so that you can knock them down." Suppose you are selling a computer-controlled liquid chromatography system. Your conclusion might be a statement that the particular model you are selling is the ideal system because it has an auto-sampler, an easy-to-use data handling system, and the industry's most reliable pump. Now you have three supporting points for the body of your talk (auto-sampler, data system, pump). And at this point you can design the "pin-setting" introduction: "The ideal liquid chromatography system should (1) make sample handling easy, (2) process the data efficiently, and (3) provide reliable pumping operation. Happily (and not just coincidentally), the system you are selling will meet all of the criteria of the ideal system.

The same approach can be used in persuading or in "selling" your *ideas*. Imagine you want to convince your audience that it is important to support research into bacteria which inhabit Antarctic penguin nesting areas. What could you use for a conclusion? "It is important for the National Science Foundation to support this research because . . ." Now you have to come up with some good reasons. Here are a few possibilities: "It is important for the National Science Foundation to support this research because (1) it will lead to a better understanding of organisms which can thrive in low temperatures, (2) it will help us understand how bacteria contribute to the ecosystem in which penguins live, and (3) it will help us understand the fragile environment of the endangered whiffle-beak penguins." You can then build the body of the talk around these reasons. Your introduction should get the audience's attention and interest them in your subject. In this example, the introduction could involve the tragic fate of the whiffle-beaks, the rather unusual appearance of penguins, or the mystery of why bacteria and birds should live in an environment which (to us, at least) seems quite hostile.

Storyboards

You may prefer the storyboard approach if you like to think visually. Also, if you have many points to cover and you are not sure how they fit together and what order to put them in, the storyboard could be the answer. And, as Thomas Leech points out, this is a good method for planning and organizing visual aids.

You can use index cards, sheets of paper, or sticky notes as the "boards." Initially you just begin writing down your ideas, one per "board." This corresponds to the "creative" phase we spoke of earlier. Don't worry about editing or organizing yet, just focus on capturing every possible supporting point, anecdote, illustration, and experimental result which might become part of your presentation. Then, when you have a stack of "boards," lay them out on a table or on the floor, stick them to your filing cabinet, put them on the wall or onto a flip chart. Think about how you wish to sort them. What order should they be in? Can you put related ones together? If you think of additional points which should be made, add more "boards."

At this stage, you can start to be more critical. Do all of your points relate directly to your main message? Are there smooth transitions from one point to the next? Is there some additional supporting information which you need to look for? Are there parts of the talk where you have *too much* material and you need to do some editing? One of the advantages of the storyboard approach is that you can easily try out different ways of organizing your material just by rearranging the "boards." Adding and subtracting material can be done easily, too. This is an especially good approach to use if you are preparing material for a supervisor who isn't quite sure what he or she wants.

Revising and refining your talk

After you have assembled your ideas and have put them into some sort of order it is time to refine your material. Writers are familiar with (and usually dread) the revision process. It's not as exciting as the "creative" phase of preparing a talk. But the revisions make the difference between a presentation which seems as if it were thrown together in the cab on the way from the airport and one which looks, sounds and feels professional. This is difficult and sometimes tedious work, but it pays off in a presentation which earns you the respect and admiration of your listeners. We will discuss three components: *flow*, "*zing*," and *timing*. Consider each of these as you refine your presentation.

Flow

If your talk flows smoothly from one point to the next you will come across as a well-prepared speaker. Now that you have some sort of outline in place there are ways to evaluate whether all of the ideas that you assembled flow smoothly. This is often the time when you notice how important the transitions are.

One way to make sure that your talk has a smooth, logical flow of thoughts is to rewrite your outline using a *complete sentence* for each point. This forces you to get a little more specific with your thoughts. Instead of having a point which is simply labeled "Efficiency," you have to compose a sentence which indicates what you plan to say about efficiency. When you do this, you may find that you need to do a little more work in one area or another. Make note of points where you need to collect more information or find answers to specific questions.

The other way to check for flow is to *talk through* your presentation. It is important that you do this aloud, and not just in your mind. Points with which you are intimately familiar may sound perfectly logical if you think through them in your mind, but when you have to express them aloud, in words, you discover places where you have to search for a missing word. You find ideas which need a more detailed explanation than you had anticipated. Make notes as you go along in order to keep track of things you need to look up or questions you need to address.

Whichever method you choose, go through the presentation several times. First go through your outline looking for a smooth, logical flow of thoughts. If there are rough spots, what kinds of transitions would help? Is there something missing which would help bridge from one thought to the next? Is there extraneous material which gets in the way of your flow? Go through a second time, asking yourself if each part of the talk relates directly to your main message. If so, is it obvious to the listener how it relates? If not, why is it there? If you have made very many changes at this point go through your outline yet another time to be sure that the flow is still there.

This is a good time to sit down with a colleague, mentor, supervisor, or friend and discuss your outline. Explain what your main message is to be, how you plan to support that message, and what points you plan to cover in your presentation. Ask for feedback about how smoothly the ideas flow and about how clearly the information is conveyed. Once again, make notes about how the talk can be improved, and revise one more time.

"Zing"

What distinguishes a great talk from a good one? Richard Roberts, who won the Nobel Prize in Medicine, certainly knows enough technical material to talk for days. But he gives an excellent 45-minute talk on his work without discussing a single detailed experimental procedure. He speaks in broad terms about RNA structure and why he finds it exciting to study this topic. He gives examples of complex phenomena which can be more clearly understood in terms of RNA structure. And his talk is peppered with *stories* about discoveries which he and his colleagues have made concerning RNA structure. He doesn't go into detail about the solvent conditions which ultimately led to the growth of an important crystal; he talks about the struggles, the attitudes, and the feelings of the graduate student who ultimately succeeded in growing an especially important crystal. If you want to know how to grow the crystal, you should look in the scientific literature for one of Dr Roberts's papers. If you want to feel the excitement of scientific research, you should go to hear a Rich Roberts seminar. The *stories* bring the science to life.

You can do exactly the same thing. Go through your outline once again, this time looking for places where a story would bring the subject to life. Look for places where a good analogy would clarify your point. Look for places where you can personalize your talk by telling why *you* are excited about the topic. Did you make a mistake in the course of your study which led you to discover something new or see something in a different way? Tell us about it! It makes you into a real, live human being, and then we can relate to you.

Timing

For scientists, just as for comedians, timing is critical. When you speak on a technical topic, you are the expert. It is neither possible nor desirable for you to transform your listeners into clones of you, with all of the knowledge you possess on the subject. After all, it took you a long time to learn all you know, and you don't have that much time to speak. This means you have to be selective in what you talk about – don't even *attempt* to tell them everything you know. You have to decide what is reasonable and important to cover within the time allotted to you.

First, be realistic about the time available. If you are speaking during a one-hour seminar period, allow for the fact that these programs frequently start five minutes late. Now you have only 55 minutes. And the person who invited you to speak may spend a couple of minutes introducing you. Is there to be a question-and-answer period? You may only have 45 minutes of that hour to work with. Are you speaking as part of a tightly structured program, such as a series of 20-minute talks? If so, it is imperative for you to stay within your time limit. In such programs, if each speaker runs five minutes over, by the end of the program the schedule is wrecked and the audience has lost its patience. Again, you may have to set aside a minute for introductions and a couple of minutes for questions. Even if you are a professor in a large lecture hall, the master of your auditorium for 50 minutes, you should allow a few minutes in case of microphone problems, lighting difficulties, or the occasional question.

Talk through your presentation (aloud!) yet another time, this time with the clock running. How long did it take? How much of your time was spent on the introduction, the body, the conclusion? If necessary, you may have to revise your outline yet another time. Most speakers find that they have too much material. If this is the case, how can you shorten your talk? Do you need to select a more narrowly focused topic? Do you have too many supporting points? A few strong points will make a better impression than an endless list of weaker ones. Are you including too much detail? In a patent or a scientific publication, you are expected to provide enough detail so that some one "skilled in the art" could reproduce your experiment; this is not a requirement or even a desirable goal for speeches. Leave out the detailed technical procedures.

Timing is also important because your audience comes to hear you with some expectations. For example, if the seminar hour is from 2 p.m. to 3 p.m., people expect that they will be out of the room at 3 p.m. If you aren't even close to a conclusion at 2:55 and there is to be a question-and-answer period following the talk, you can be sure that some of your listeners will start to become impatient. If you are still talking at 3:05, most of the (former) listeners are now thinking about what they had planned to do at 3 p.m., or are wondering how to sneak out of the room without being noticed. Robert Anholt describes this problem in terms of the amount of "listener energy" which is brought to the event. Each listener comes prepared to invest a certain amount of time and energy in your talk. If you exceed that energy budget you will lose your audience. And this will happen at the worst possible time: the conclusion, which is where you should be bringing all of the pieces together and cementing your key message in the listeners' minds.

Plan ahead for the possibility that your talk may have to be cut short. Suppose that a late start, a fire drill, or a burned-out projector bulb forces you to cut some material from your presentation. What would you leave out? Do not cut down on your conclusion, since this should be a carefully crafted finish which drives home your take-home message. Instead, decide what details could be condensed, omitted, or glossed over in the body of your talk.

Finally, watch the clock from time to time during your talk. If there isn't a clock visible to you, bring along a watch with a large, easy-to-read face. You should have a pretty good idea of how long each section of your talk takes, especially the conclusion. Then, no matter what, adjust the length of the body of your talk so that you preserve the time needed for your conclusion.

If you decide to omit some material, do not feel compelled to announce this to your audience. This would detract from the smooth flow of your presentation. The audience will not know what you intended to say, so they will not notice what you choose to leave out.

Summary

You have now chosen a formula (introduction–body–conclusion, question and answer, AIDA, the ho-hum method, or motivated sequence) that puts your presentation all together. Next you have skillfully collected and arranged your ideas and information around your key message, using a method such as *outlining, mind-mapping*, "*start at the end*" or *storyboards*. Finally, by giving attention to transitions and "flow," "zing" and "timing," your good talk has been revised and refined into a *great* talk.

Some key messages from this chapter

- *Make your **key message** the centerpiece around which your talk is constructed. The key message should be in the introduction of your talk, the body of the talk should be built around that key message, and the conclusion should serve to reinforce the key message.*
- *Collect and arrange your ideas in two distinct stages: a **creative** phase, followed by a **critical** (editing) phase.*
- *Talk through your presentation aloud, not just in your mind, to be sure that it flows smoothly and fits into the allotted time.*
- *Put life and personality into your talk. Include stories about the people involved, their experiences, and their feelings.*

Exercises

1 Select a scientific or technical topic with which you are familiar. Formulate a key message around that topic. How would you develop this key message in an introduction–body–conclusion format? Can you frame it in a question and answer format? How could you adapt it to the AIDA, ho-hum, or motivated sequence formulas?

2 Have you previously used the outlining, mind-mapping, start-at-the-end, or storyboard methods in organizing your material? For your selected topic and key message, use a method you have *not* previously tried, to develop the framework for a presentation.

3 The next time you attend a lecture or seminar, see whether the speaker has used good transitions to move from one point to the next. Did the speaker incorporate any real-life experiences in the talk?

Chapter 3

Visual aids

Technically oriented speakers often begin work on their presentations by making their visual aids. Maybe this is because your visual aids are the easiest part of your talk to improve. With just a little effort you can make a striking difference in your presentation. Nevertheless, preparation of your visual aids should be done *after* you have carefully planned what you want to tell your audience. In this chapter we will discuss four aspects of visual aids.

1 What should and should not be in a visual aid
2 Types of visual aids
3 Preparing the visual aids
4 Using the visual aids

What should and should not be in a visual aid

The visual aid is not the main event – the role of the visual aid is to *illustrate* or *emphasize* what you say. Good visual aids can increase the audience's retention of what you say. It is not necessary (or even desirable) to have a visual aid for every point you make. If there are too many visuals, they lose their impact and *nothing* is emphasized. It seems as though you are constantly shuffling things, and the visual aids get more attention than your words.

The visual aids should not serve as your Teleprompter or script, either. Many speakers fall into the bad habit of using their visual aids as speaking notes. The screen is filled with the speaker's outline or key sentences, and the speaker reads to the audience. If your notes are on the screen, you will spend far too much time looking at the screen instead of your audience. Besides, the audience will read ahead instead of listening to you. And a screen full of text has one more adverse effect: you cannot make eye contact with people whose eyes are riveted to the projection screen. If you just have a few key-words on the screen, people will listen to find out why you put them there. If you need speaking notes, they should be separate from your visual aids.

Finally, a bad visual aid is worse than no visual aid at all. If you feel compelled to apologize for a visual aid, *leave it out*. Apologizing will call everyone's attention to a negative aspect of your presenta-tion. Your audience may get the feeling you didn't care enough to make a better figure for them.

Types of visual aids

In choosing appropriate visual aids you must take several factors into account. How big is the room? How many people are in your audience? What is the goal of this presentation? How much time, money, and effort can you afford to put into this presentation? There are many kinds of visual aids to choose from, and you must decide which will best fit your circumstances. Your choices include:

- Overhead transparencies
- 35 mm slides
- Flip charts
- Blackboard or marker board
- Video
- Computer projection
- Handouts
- Models and products

Overhead transparencies

Overhead transparencies (also referred to as viewgraphs or acetates) are probably the most versatile of visual aids. They are very easy to make, since photocopying machines and printers can be used for this purpose. Overheads are inexpensive enough to use just once.

Overheads work well in small conference rooms as well as in fairly large auditoriums. The projector is in the front of the room, so you can easily control the projection as you speak. One of the major advantages of overheads is that you can use them without darkening the room very much. As we will see in a later chapter, it is important to be able to see the faces of the people you are speaking to so that you will be able to tell how well they are following your presentation. The audience needs to be able to see your facial expression and your body language as well.

On the downside, overheads can be annoying to the presenter during the talk. They are sometimes slippery, and your stack of transparencies could accidentally slip onto the floor. At other times they seem to be charged with static electricity, and are difficult to separate. If your transparency has a backing sheet attached to help it feed through the copier or printer, it's a good idea to remove this sheet ahead of time rather than fumble with it during your presentation. Transparencies are also prone to show wear and tear easily. Handle them carefully during rehearsals. If you plan to use them more than once, protect them with frames or page protectors designed for this purpose (you can find these at an office supply store). The frames, usually white cardboard, have the added benefit of providing a place on which you can write notes to remind yourself of specific points you wish to make for that overhead.

You can effectively add color to your overheads, either with a color printer or with colored marking pens. Make a few tests to be sure your color printer or colored markers make transparencies which project well.

Overheads also allow you to be quite flexible in your presentation. You may draw or write on your transparencies as you speak, or in response to questions. If you bring along some blank transparencies and markers you can make additional diagrams or illustrations on the spur of the moment. When you are writing or drawing on transparencies watch for the following:

- Take your time – hurrying leads to scribbling, which hinders communication
- Print clearly, using large letters
- Draw simply, using a few bold lines
- Use markers which project clearly and which write on the kind of plastic you are using – water-based markers sometimes "bead up" on the plastic

Transparencies lend themselves readily to the "overlay" technique. You can start with a fairly simple diagram, then overlay another transparency which adds detail. This can be an effective way to illustrate something which is very complex. Figure 3.1

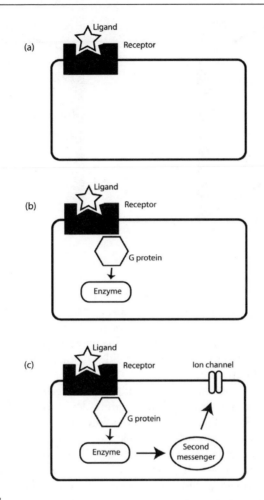

Figure 3.1

shows an example in which we use overlays to illustrate a five-step sequence of events. We begin in (a) with the first step, the interaction of a ligand with a receptor on the surface of a cell. In (b), we show the next two steps: receptor activation of a G protein and G protein activation of an enzyme inside the cell. Finally, in (c), we indicate production of a second messenger which activates an ion channel. If we had started with (c), it might have been too complex an illustration.

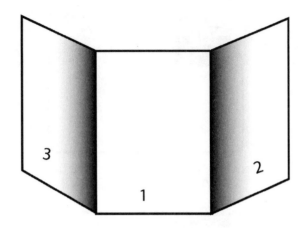

Figure 3.2

Spend some time planning and practicing if you are going to do overlays. Two overlays on one transparency is a practical limit. If it is hard to line up the overlay properly, you should consider whether the drawing is too detailed. One way to make the alignment easier is to tape the overlays onto the sides of the main transparency, as shown in Figure 3.2.

Closely related to the overlay method is the technique of starting with a fairly simple overhead and adding detail to it with marking pens as you speak. Figure 3.3 is taken from a lecture on porphyrin structures. Part (a) shows the basic porphyrin ring structure. It would take too much time to draw the whole ring for each porphyrin to be discussed, so several copies of this core structure transparency are made in advance. Different biologically important porphyrins have different substitution patterns around the core structure, and one of these is illustrated in part (b). By adding the substituents during the lecture, the characteristics of different porphyrins are emphasized. Students also are reminded that the core structure is the same throughout the series.

Another technique which may be effective if used properly is to cover part of your transparency with a sheet of paper to control how much is revealed. As you progress, you reveal more of the transparency until you get a complete picture. This can work well with a bullet list, where the last item is to be a surprise, for instance. You can slide an ordinary sheet of paper down to reveal one point

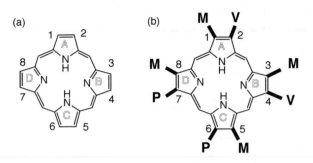

Detail can be added during your talk, to highlight important features. (a) The core structure for a whole series of porphyrinas is the starting point for the transparency. (b) During the lecture, the side chain pattern is added, stressing the important features of the particular porphyrin under consideration.

Figure 3.3

after another, or you can cover with a series of Post-it Notes, which stay in place while you talk and are quite easy to remove.

Figure 3.4 shows an instance in which this "unveiling" technique is useful. The amino acid methionine is made by transferring a carbon atom from serine onto tetrahydrofolate, then to vitamin B_{12}, and finally to homocysteine. If you show all three of the reactions at once you may overwhelm your listeners. If you make three separate transparencies your listeners may lose sight of the overall scheme. A sheet of paper can be used to cover the second and third reactions while you discuss the first reaction. You can then slide the paper down to reveal the second reaction. Finally, you can remove the paper to show the third reaction.

Be careful not to overuse the "unveiling" technique. Some people are very annoyed to think that you are hiding something from them. And if you find yourself using it often, it may mean that you are putting too many things on one overhead. It might be better to split the material onto two or more different overheads.

Slides

Slides (35 mm) can be the most polished and professional-looking visual aids. The changing of slides is usually smoother than changing transparencies. And slides are more durable than transparencies, which may be an issue if you will be re-using them several times. Slides work well in very large rooms. On the other hand, fan noise

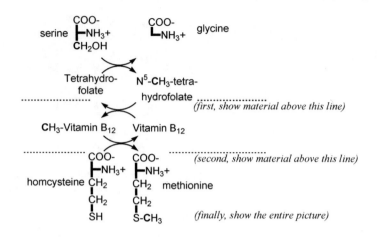

Figure 3.4

from the projector may become a distraction in a small conference room.

Slides generally require a darker room, especially if your slides do not have high contrast. This cuts down on your ability to make eye contact with your audience, and it makes it more difficult for your listeners to see your facial expressions and gestures.

When using slides, find out in advance whether you will be changing your own slides or asking someone else to change them. Changing your own is less obtrusive than having to say "Next slide, please" throughout your talk. If you will be using a particular slide more than once, make additional copies of it. Shuffling back through several slides is distracting, and the reverse button seems to be the least reliable feature on most slide projectors.

Preview your slides to be sure they are inserted properly. There are eight ways to put a slide into the projector, and seven of them are wrong – you don't want your slides to be projected sideways, upside-down, backwards, or upside-down and backwards. If you are bringing your own carousel, use the 80-slide model; the 140-slide model is more prone to jamming.

Flip charts

Flip charts are especially common in corporate conference rooms. You get an easel with a giant pad of paper, and one or more markers.

You may write as you go, or you may prepare your flip chart in advance. In either case, you should give some thought and planning to what will go on each page. As with all visual aids, you should write down only keywords, and keep diagrams simple. Print clearly, using large letters (at least 2 in. [5 cm]). Draw simply and clearly, using bold lines.

Using the flip chart takes some practice and some attention to set up. First, be sure the chart is situated so that everyone has a clear view. If necessary, move the chart or ask your viewers to move to a place where they can see. When you are preparing the chart in advance, you may wish to alternate blank pages with the pages you use. This enables you to display a blank page during those times when a visual is not needed, so that all attention is on your message. Use blank pages in between if your markers bleed through onto the next page.

If you are writing on the chart as you go, be sure you are not speaking to the chart. Stop talking, write your keywords, then turn to the audience and resume speaking. At first this may seem awkward, so practice it until you are comfortable with it. While you are practicing, check to be sure you stand far enough away so that everyone can see. And be sure to give your audience time to absorb the contents of a page before you flip to the next one. If there is a diagram or sentence which they need to get, be sure you allow them an appropriate amount of time.

Flip charts are particularly well suited for "idea sessions" or other occasions when you want to gain audience participation. You can raise a question, then start recording responses on the chart. As you fill a page, you can tear it off and tape it to the wall with masking tape, then continue onto another sheet. In this type of situation, consider whether you wish to be the "scribe" or whether you want to assign that role to another person.

The chart can also serve as a way to handle issues that would take too much time to cover during your presentation session. Some people refer to this technique as moving an issue or topic to "the parking lot." Rather than let your meeting get sidetracked by a discussion of peripheral topics, you or your "scribe" can record the issues on a separate page. You can also attach the names of those responsible for handling these issues, expected actions, and timetables for follow-up action.

Blackboards and marker boards

Blackboards are still used in many classroom lectures. Marker boards are a common tool for less formal discussions and meetings. In both kinds of settings it is important to write with large, clear letters, and to draw simple diagrams which are easy to follow.

Much of the advice for flip charts applies to blackboards and marker boards as well. Since you usually won't be able to put up your material in advance, as you could on a flip chart, you have to do some careful planning. Practice so you will know exactly what you want to put on the board and how much time it will take. Write, then turn and talk to the people; boards are not good listeners. Make sure you allow people time to see and absorb what you have put on the board before you erase it. Finally, watch where you stand so that you aren't blocking anyone's view.

Video

First, be sure there is a good reason for using video in your presentation, because this is one of the most complicated visual aids. The process of turning on a VCR and monitor or projector for showing a video can be disruptive to your presentation, since the equipment often needs time to warm up. Attention must be given to how well the sound and picture will project in your particular setting. Monitors can only be seen clearly for a fairly short distance, and projection equipment sometimes produces fuzzy, faded-out images. Keep the video material as brief as possible. If your video is more than a few minutes long, your audience will tend to tune out and lose the flow of your talk.

Suitable applications for using a video might include something where motion needs to be shown, or for a demonstration which is difficult or costly to replicate. For example, video could be the most effective way to show microscopic crystal growth, using time-lapse photography. Occasionally, especially in the case of corporate presentations, you may choose to hire professionals to produce your video. Obviously this approach could cost thousands of dollars, but it has the benefit of providing experienced camera people and experienced advice on your presentation, your speaking style, the props you might use, the room settings and even your choice of clothing color.

When preparing your own video, plan carefully. Be sure the tape is carefully edited to show just what you want. Preview the video in the room you will be using, on the equipment you will be using, to make sure everyone will be able to see (and hear, if there is to be a soundtrack). Practice your narration so that it matches the timing and content of the video. Test all equipment several times, including moments before your presentation if possible. Be sure you know how to operate all of the components of the system. Make certain that your videotape is cued up to the proper starting point. Everyone hates to miss the beginning of a movie; conversely, people will become impatient if they must sit through much blank tape before the action starts.

Computer projection

It is now possible to project for an audience anything you see on your computer screen, enabling you to bypass the transfer of your visual aids onto transparencies or slides. With a portable computer, you can take some very elaborate computer graphics with you and show them to an audience using monitors or projection equipment. You can make changes to your presentation at the last minute, or even while you are in the midst of the presentation. The biggest limitation is the relatively low resolution of some computer displays; it can be substantially inferior to slides or overheads. Projection onto a large screen makes the low resolution even more obvious. As in the case of video, you must give consideration to how well each member of the audience can see your visual aids.

The most careful preparation and practice is required if you decide to display directly from a computer. Test all equipment thoroughly several times, including right before your presentation. If you are using someone else's computer equipment make sure that the hardware, operating system, and software are compatible with what you used to prepare your materials. Make sure you know which buttons on the keyboard or mouse move you around in your presentation, without accidentally making your screen shrink in size or close. Turn off your screensaver, or else it will activate at an inopportune time. Also make sure you know where all of the necessary files are on your computer. It would be a good idea to have a backup copy of any necessary files on a separate disk, just in case a file becomes damaged. Many speakers still carry a set of overhead transparencies to cover the possibility of computer crashes.

Models and products

Sometimes it is most effective to use a physical model or the actual item you are discussing. In a lecture about the sense of smell, you might uncork a bottle of something fragrant; if you are talking about the densities of different gases, you might bring along a helium balloon. If you are selling or demonstrating something, consider whether you can bring it along (or perhaps a model, if you are selling something the size of a space shuttle!). You can be quite creative in your choice of models – for example, you might use two cans and a string in a discussion of computer networks. A very unconventional model can make your talk quite memorable – the important point is to make sure that whatever you use is visible to everyone in the room. If you decide that an effective use of your model or product is to hand it to the audience to pass around, make sure the item is sturdy enough to take all the handling. If there is any chance that the item could break, leak, or soil people's hands or clothing, warn them in advance, and have paper towels or napkins available.

Handouts

A handout leaves the audience with something concrete to remember you by. You can include more detail on a handout than you could on a slide. And you have better control of what message the listeners take away from your talk – *you* write it down, so it doesn't get filtered through someone else's ears, brain, or hand. Check to see that the handout clearly spells out your key message. As with all visual aids, proofread for spelling and factual accuracy. Keep the handout as simple as possible. You don't want your message to be lost in a sea of details. Also, make certain that the handout contains appropriate information so that your listener will be able to get in touch with you if there is further interest at a later date.

But handouts can be distracting – people may be reading instead of listening. You must consider when to hand out the handout, and how to distribute it. If you pass them out *before* your talk, people will read ahead, and they may read instead of listening. This up-front distribution usually works best if your handout just provides a framework on which the listeners can take notes. If you are distributing your handout at the end of the talk, it can be more detailed. And if you plan to hand it out *during* your presentation, you may wish to enlist one or more of your listeners to help in the distribution so that it proceeds quickly and does not excessively disrupt your talk. One effective way to control the timing of handout distribution is to put the material in envelopes which are taped under the chairs prior to the audience's arrival.

Bring enough handouts. Better yet, bring too many. If some people are left out, you will have antagonized a portion of your audience before you begin.

Preparing the visual aids

The first consideration in designing a visual aid is so simple that it sounds trivial: present *one* idea per slide. But watch other speakers. See how often a visual aid is loaded with two, or three, or even more points. If you have more than one idea on a visual, you risk confusing or distracting the audience, and your visual aid may become too complex. You also tempt people to look ahead and start asking questions about a topic you have not yet covered. Evaluate each visual aid with these two questions:

- What idea does this visual illustrate?
- Does this visual aid directly support my "key message"?

The amount of information which you can comprehend on a printed page or on a computer screen is far too much for a visual aid. Keep your visual aids as simple as possible. When your transparencies contain too much text, too many details, or things which are too tiny to see clearly, you no longer have a visual aid, you have a visual *hindrance*. Use keywords only, and use LARGE print.

Presentation software makes it easy – too easy?

There are numerous computer programs designed to help in preparing presentations. They make it easy to add backgrounds, borders, different fonts and different colors. In fact, they make it too easy. These programs tempt us with long lists of fonts, ranging from Gothic to Cutesy. Resist the temptation! Select one clear, clean font and use it consistently. On a written page containing a great deal of text, a font such as Times New Roman (with serifs) may be easiest to read, so this would be a good choice for handouts. For slides and transparencies, a sans serif font such as **Helvetica** projects more clearly (see the box below). For emphasis, you may choose any *one* of the following: **boldface**, *italic*, a different color, or <u>underline</u>.

This is the Times font, which has serifs. It is good for text on the printed page.	This is the Helvetica font. It is a good choice for the presentation of graphics.

The availability of 256 million colors also forces us to make some choices. The first time you try a presentation software program go ahead and experiment with the colors. Play with a dozen text colors on one slide; add baroque borders and rainbow backgrounds. While these look great on the computer monitor, they often translate into absolutely wretched slides which can only be seen in a totally darkened room. So when you are ready to make visual aids for your presentation, select a fairly simple background, border, and color scheme, and use them consistently. The most important factor is contrast. Black text on a white background provides maximum contrast; white text on a black background has equal contrast, but it will give you less light in the room, so that it is harder to see your audience. If you choose to use colors, think in terms of the contrast between the colors you choose. Yellow on a very dark blue background is quite good. Black on a light blue background can be problematic, depending on how dark your printer or photographer makes the blue. You can use a third color for emphasis. If you go beyond three colors, make sure there is a *very* good reason for doing so.

Colors convey subtle implications in addition to providing contrast. Red, yellow, and orange are "hot" colors which may be used to indicate action. Blue, green, and purple are "cool" colors which connote trust.

Layout

One of the choices you must make when using presentation software is whether to use landscape or portrait layout (Figure 3.5). When you use 35 mm slides, *always* use landscape (horizontal) layout rather than portrait. Many lecture rooms are set up so as to fill the screen with a landscape-style slide, so when one of your slides is in

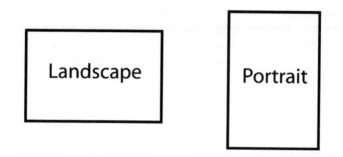

Figure 3.5

portrait mode to show a giraffe eating leaves from a tall tree, the leaves and the head will be spread across the ceiling. Here is what happens next: a helpful person in the back of the room feels compelled to tilt the slide projector to bring the giraffe's head down onto the screen, and the ensuing irregular motion of the projector begins to make your audience seasick. Magazines, books, and other found objects are used to adjust the projector position. And now the bottoms of all successive slides are cut off!

Using text on your visual aids

Only in rare circumstances should you put a complete sentence on a visual aid. Delivering sentences is the job of the speaker, after all. If your words exactly match those on the screen, listeners think you are reading it, and if you have to read it, listeners think that you don't really know it. Furthermore, if your words don't exactly match the sentence on the screen, the incongruity will grate in the listener's mind.

It is very easy to fall into the bad habit of using visual aids as a script. When you do this, you spend far too much of your time facing the screen rather than the audience. People miss much of the expressiveness of your face and begin to feel that you are not really speaking to them. They can read much faster than you can speak, so they move ahead of you and then become distracted while waiting for you to catch up. Visual aids which show text should generally contain only keywords. If you write sentences or paragraphs, your audience will inexorably be drawn into *reading* instead of *listening*. Bullet charts are a good way to help your audience quickly see your key points and put them into context. The four-by-four rule is a good guideline when putting text onto a visual aid: use no more than four lines of text per slide, and no more than four words per line. This allows you to use a large font so that everyone will be able to see. Just put a few keywords in your visual aid, not the complete text of your presentation. If you need to have notes for your talk, these should be completely separate from your visual aids.

Graphs and drawings

The reason for using a graph or drawing is to illustrate or clarify something. Usually a very simple, schematic drawing will do quite nicely – the fewer lines the better. The amount of detail which works well on a printed page or on a computer screen is often far too much for a visual aid. Details which are important in a publication may safely be omitted from your visual aid. For example, on a printed page it may be important to extensively label the axes; in a visual aid you just want to convey the "big picture." As an example, look at graph (a) in Figure 3.6. In print this graph is quite readable, but when it is projected onto a screen there are too many lines and the numbers are much too small. In (b), we have simplified the graph, made the lines bolder, and replaced the legend with much larger labels. If your real goal were to show that government support of health research declined (on a percentage basis) over this time period, you could use an even simpler graph, as shown in (c).

When you are using a graph or a drawing in your visual aid, make all of the lines about four times as thick as you would when printing onto a sheet of paper. Thin lines disappear from the screen if the focus is even a little fuzzy. Also, a few bold lines will make a much stronger impression than many fine ones. And if you use thick lines, it will help you remember to use the minimum number of lines necessary to illustrate your point.

It may take a fair amount of time to look at a table of numerical data and understand what is going on. Graphs let you convert this numerical data into pictorial forms which can have much more immediate impact. Pie charts can quickly convey percentages or fractions of a whole subject. How often does glutamate occur in proteins? What is the most abundant amino acid in our protein database? Table 3.1 tells us the numbers, but the pie graph (see Figure 3.7) can have a much greater visual impact.

(a)

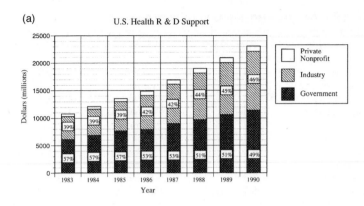

U.S. Health R & D Support

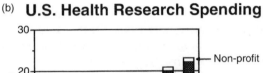

(b) **U.S. Health Research Spending**

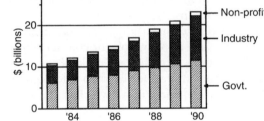

(c)

U.S. Health Research Spending

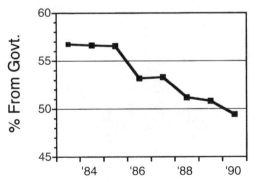

Figure 3.6

Table 3.1 Amino acid frequency in a protein database

Amino acid	Percentage	Amino acid	Percentage
Alanine	8.3	Leucine	9.0
Arginine	5.7	Lysine	5.7
Asparagine	4.4	Methionine	2.4
Aspartate	5.3	Phenylalanine	3.9
Cysteine	1.7	Proline	5.1
Glutamate	6.2	Serine	6.9
Glutamine	4.0	Threonine	5.8
Glycine	7.2	Tryptophan	1.3
Histidine	2.3	Tyrosine	3.2
Isoleucine	5.2	Valine	6.6

Bar graphs are well suited to the representation of one-dimensional data and simple comparisons. See the "Research Spending" graphs (Figure 3.6) for an example. For two-dimensional data and correlations, you may use scatter plots or line graphs, as illustrated in Figure 3.8. Three-dimensional data may require more complex representations such as 3D graphs or contour plots.

As with graphs, illustrations should be as simple as possible. Often a schematic diagram is much more effective than a detailed drawing or photograph. Whenever you add a detail which is not required to

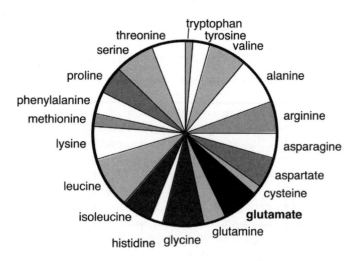

Figure 3.7

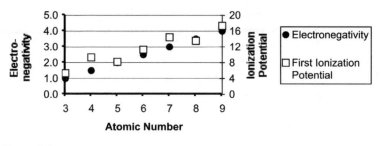

Figure 3.8

support your main message you run the risk of distracting people from your real point.

Using the visual aids

Before using your visual aids in an actual presentation, project them onto a screen. Look for spelling, grammatical, and typographical errors. A spelling error seems much worse when it is projected onto a 30-foot screen! If you aren't very good at proofreading and spelling, enlist the help of someone who has a good critical eye.

If you need to show a particular visual aid more than once, make additional copies of it. Shuffling through a pile of transparencies is distracting and makes you look unprepared. Backing up through a series of slides in a projector tray is risky business, since not all projectors have a reverse button, and many of those which have one do not work properly.

Pre-talk preparation should include peeling any backing materials off of your overheads; making sure that slides project right-side up and that they can be focused properly; ensuring that pens/markers/ chalk are available and in working order; ensuring that flip charts have plenty of paper; knowing where the spare projector bulbs are located. Preview your visual aids on screen, preferably in the room you will be using. Check the size and clarity of all visual aids. Check the visibility throughout the room. Where will you be standing? Be certain that you don't block the listeners' view. Sit in the *back* of the room and see whether each image is clearly visible and understandable. Give some thought to how you will handle your presentation in case something goes wrong. If you are using video, computers, or other high-tech visual aids, test them *thoroughly* and have backup plans.

No matter what kinds of visual aids you choose, you should practice your talk while using them to be sure they fit with your verbal message. Then practice the whole presentation with your visual aids several more times, just to be sure. Practice so thoroughly that your visual aids become a fully integrated part of the total presentation. If you do this, people will notice how impressively you delivered your message rather than how pretty your pictures were. That's your real objective, isn't it?

When it comes to show time be sure you have your visual aids under control. You can increase your *visual presence* (the sense that you, the speaker, are in control) by actively controlling what the audience sees at all times. We are often too distracted or too careless to do this – we put up a slide and leave it up long after we have made the point on the slide, or we put the next slide up before we are ready to discuss it. Each visual aid should be displayed *only* while it is relevant to what you are saying. At all other times you should have *nothing* displayed, because it will only distract your listeners from hearing your message. This may mean we have to put some blank slides into the carousel, or we may have to remember to take a transparency off without reflexively putting the next one on. There does not have to be something on the screen at all times. You may turn off the projector if it is not going to be used for a substantial amount of time, but don't turn it off–on–off–on–off too frequently, as this would also be distracting.

Face your audience throughout your talk. In an ideal world, perhaps no visual aid would be so complicated that you would have to point to a specific part of it. In reality, though, we sometimes have to point. Your pointer may be your hand, a stick, an old car radio antenna, or a laser beam. Learn to use the touch–turn–talk technique. Your mission is to point, then turn back toward your audience and speak *to the people*, not to the item you are pointing to. You may have to practice doing this many times before you do it naturally. This seems to be one of the most difficult things to master for people giving technical presentations. Don't give up. If you learn to point, turn, and talk, you will distinguish yourself from 99 percent of your peers.

If you are given the choice of a laser pointer or a stick, *please* pick the low-tech stick. It is much more difficult to point steadily with a little flashlight than with a substantial stick. The jumpy red dot can be both annoying and distracting. If you are one of those people who makes endless circles with the red dot, please stop immediately – you make us dizzy!

When you are using an overhead projector, you may point at the screen, or you may use a pencil to point on the transparency. If you choose the latter, *practice* in order to be sure you are not blocking the screen with your hand, body, or head. When you are not using the pointer, put it down – don't play with it.

There is one more thing you can do to minimize distractions from your visual aids: select one kind of visual aid and stick with it. Many people are tempted to take the 35 mm slides from a previous talk, then add in a few overheads to update it. This creates discontinuity every time the slide projector must be turned off and the overhead projector turned on (or vice versa). You may get away with adding a few overheads at the end of a slide presentation, but multiple changes really should be avoided.

Summary

When you trade in your too-tiny pictures and too-busy text for some bold, clear graphics, your presentation will be visibly improved. For each visual aid you have planned, ask these questions:

- Why is it there?
- What does it show?
- Does it show this clearly, even for people in the back row?
- Does it support the key message?
- Is there anything there which doesn't need to be there?
- When will it be shown? When will it be removed?

Some key messages from this chapter

- *Plan your talk first, **then** decide what visual aids you will need.*
- *The visual aids are there to illustrate or emphasize what you say – they are **not** the main event.*
- *Present **one** topic per visual aid.*
- *Use a minimal amount of text, in a large, clear font.*
- *Keep figures as simple as possible.*
- *Practice with your visual aids. Check all equipment before your presentation.*

Exercise

Prepare a brief talk on a topic with which you are very familiar. Then answer the following questions:

- What visual aids would I use if I were presenting this talk with overheads, slides, or computer projection?
- How would I illustrate this talk on a blackboard or marker board?
- What kind of handouts would I use with this talk?

Box 3.1 Advantages and disadvantages of different kinds of visual aids

Visual aid	Advantages	Disadvantages
Transparencies	Easy to prepare Easy to modify or create Keep room lights up	Hard to align and center Static electricity, sticks together A stack can slide onto floor
35 mm slides	Professional appearance	Harder to prepare Room must be darker Equipment can be balky
Flip charts	Good for audience participation Can tear off pages and hang them	Pens dry up Pens can have a strong smell Less portable Back to audience
Blackboard/ marker board	Good for building up diagrams	Back to audience
Video	Can show motion Can capture a difficult demo	May be difficult to see Room may be darkened
Computer display	Easy to prepare Portable	Higher risk of technical problems May be difficult to see
Models	Visual impact	May be awkward to transport
Handouts	Concrete reminder of message Can contain more detail	When to hand out? May be distracting

Chapter 4

Practice, practice, practice

The final step in preparation for your presentation is *practice*. The old adage "practice makes perfect" reminds us of the importance of rehearsal, but it may discourage those who know they will never be perfect. Instead, remember that "practice makes better," and the more you practice, the better your presentation will be. Start practicing early. Once you begin, you will find that there are visual aids which need to be modified, or missing pieces of information which you need to research. You may have to add or subtract material so that the timing comes out right. Give yourself enough time to handle these things.

Practice accomplishes several purposes. With practice, you will refine your presentation so that it flows more logically and smoothly. Practicing with your visual aids will help you to integrate them more smoothly. Practice lets you get used to a real room with real audio-visual equipment and real people listening, so that you can minimize stage fright when the time comes for you to deliver your presentation. Practice helps you fit your talk to the time allotted. And with practice you can reduce your reliance on written text or notes so that you can relate more directly to your audience.

Let the words flow

"Flow" is the smooth, logical progression of your talk. Good organization (Chapter 2) lays the foundation, but *practice* is essential in developing the flow of your talk.

When you practice, be sure to practice out loud. We are often too self-conscious to call in our friends and do the talk out loud, so we just run through the speech mentally. When we do this we miss a few things.

If you practice "in your head" it is very easy to glide over concepts which, in your mind, you may understand, but which are difficult to articulate in words. It is critical to identify these points and to work through the *specific words* you will use to explain them. Otherwise, you will find yourself in front of a group of people, fumbling for the words you need to make yourself understood.

As you practice, check to see that you are speaking in very *specific* words. Replace words like "et cetera" and "and so forth" with one or more examples; otherwise your message will become vague and diluted. For instance, instead of saying "Protease inhibition may lead to treatments for many different diseases," you could say "Protease inhibition may lead to treatments for HIV infection, arthritis, high blood pressure, and stroke." Your listeners can identify with one or more specific diseases much more readily than with the ethereal "many diseases."

When you talk through your presentation out loud you may also discover parts of the story which need to be rearranged. You may find you need to provide some background information before you can make a necessary argument. If you were writing your message for publication, a reader could go off and locate that material and then return to your paper, but this isn't possible in an oral presentation.

Another aspect of flow becomes more apparent when you practice aloud: transitions. Transitions are sentences which lead the listener from one point to the next. They tell the listener when you have completed a topic, and this helps the listener to assimilate your message in logical pieces. Here is an example: "Now that we have seen how the protease enzyme works, let's take a look at what happens when we block the activity of the enzyme." This lets people know you are through talking about how the enzyme works. Does anyone look confused? If so, you may wish to stop for a question or two. You have also signaled that you are about to jump into a new aspect of your subject. It's the oral equivalent of a subject heading on the written page. It lets people know once again in what direction you are going, and it may serve to recapture attention if someone's mind happens to be wandering.

Watch your timing

Every speaking occasion has a time allotment. At the very least, the audience comes with a time-frame in mind. Exceeding this time allotment is both inconsiderate and dangerous, as we discussed in Chapter 2. When you run beyond the real or presumed time limit you show a lack of respect for other people's time, and they may well respond with declining respect for you as a speaker.

Use your rehearsals to check the timing of your talk. Keep in mind that many speaking events do not start exactly on time; allow for about 5 minutes delay unless you *know* that the timing of the program is to be strictly regulated. You may want to set aside time at the end for questions, so you should probably plan on speaking for only 45 minutes if you have a one-hour time allotment. If you have any questions about how long you can spend speaking, work them out with your host ahead of time – make no assumptions.

What about notes?

In the beginning, use as many notes as you need. You can even read your speech if necessary. But after you have practiced a few times, replace the text with a detailed outline. Don't worry about reproducing identical wording every time. You should work toward being able to look at a topic on your outline and then talk about it easily – it should sound almost conversational. When you see a particular keyword, it should remind you of the particular point you wish to make about that topic, and the exact words you use are not especially important. After a few times through with the detailed outline, substitute a more concise outline. Finally, use a brief outline containing only keywords. The goal is *not* to eventually recite the speech from memory, but to wean yourself away from the notes, allowing you to focus more of your attention on your *listeners*.

Let us remind you once again that you should not use your visual aids as speaking notes. Remember, the visual aids should have only keywords which you want to reinforce in your listeners' minds. If you need speaking notes, just make up a separate set of speaking notes. Keep them in front of you so that you aren't constantly looking toward a screen and away from your audience.

Get feedback

In the beginning, you may wish to talk through the speech in an empty room. Sooner or later, though, you should ask a mentor, colleague, or friend to listen and to make constructive comments.

Some companies will bring in a consultant to prepare a presenter, especially for question and answer sessions. Objective feedback will help you to identify quickly the things you need to work on, and it will help you to know if you are making progress on these things.

What makes a good evaluator? It's not so important that this person knows your topic well. In fact, someone who is less familiar with your subject may be in a better position to know if you have explained it well. You should choose someone who has reasonably good speaking skills if possible. If you are not a native English speaker make every effort to get a native English speaker to help you with words and pronunciations. It may be much easier for you to ask your friends who speak your native language to help you out, but they may not be very helpful in identifying language problems.

Constructive evaluation can be carried out as a three-step process:

- What did you do well?
- What is the most important thing for you to improve next time?
- Where did you show particular improvement?

At the end of the chapter we have provided some guidelines and a checklist to help your colleagues evaluate your performance. To be effective, the evaluation should be honest but not cruel. Let's elaborate on those three steps.

Evaluation should begin with the things you did well. Positive reinforcement is much more effective than negative comments. Child psychologists tell us that the best way to change a child's behavior is to notice positive behavior and comment favorably on it. We aren't so different from children – we appreciate some encouragement when we do things well.

Next, the evaluation should identify the one or two most important things to improve upon. It would be discouraging to list all of your shortcomings at once, especially when you are getting started. It's better to work on one skill at a time, master it, and then move on to something else. If you work on your biggest problem first you will see rapid improvement, and it will not be long before you find yourself polishing up the finer points.

Finally, it is important to be told when you are improving. Ask your evaluator to watch out for things that have caused you problems in the past. If you are concentrating on a particular aspect of your presentation (overcoming a monotone, for instance), alert your evaluator to watch that aspect of your talk carefully. Even if it hasn't yet become one of your strengths, you need to know when you are making some progress in overcoming a difficult problem.

Practice allows you to make the *mechanical* aspects of speaking *automatic*, so that you are free to put more of your personality into the talk. Additionally, making the basic presentation skills routine will allow you the freedom to observe the crowd and adapt your talk as you go along. If you see people nodding off, you know you need to crank up your energy. If listeners look confused, invite them to ask questions before you move on. You will also find that it becomes easier to keep an eye on the clock, adjusting your presentation as you go so that you finish on time.

Integrate your visual aids

As we discussed in Chapter 3, it is important to practice working with your visual aids, whether they are overheads, slides, video, models, or something else. Pay attention to when the visual aid should be displayed and when it should be removed. Make sure each visual aid is clear and accurate, and that it supports the point you are making. Practice talking *about* your visual aids without staring at them and talking *to* them. As you practice, you may find that some of your visual aids are not necessary at all. You may also discover places in your talk where a visual aid could profitably be added.

Ask your evaluators for suggestions about how to improve your visual aids. Sometimes a fresh viewpoint is needed to identify what's wrong with a particular graph or diagram.

Your rehearsal should include ensuring that you know how to turn on equipment and adjust it. Do you know how to focus the projector, change the bulb, adjust the microphone volume, control the room lights? Extra attention should be paid to video and computer equipment. How long does it take the equipment to warm up? How do you cue up the correct starting point? What do you do if the computer crashes? If you have dealt with these issues in your rehearsals, you won't become nervous and flustered when they arise during your presentation.

Get comfortable with your setting

If it is possible to do so, practice your talk in the room you will be speaking in. Get used to the view from the stage. Familiarize yourself with the look and sound of the room. If this isn't possible, at least look at the room. When you have been invited to speak in a place where you can't visit the room ahead of time, ask your host to tell you about the setting for the talk, and practice in a similar setting.

It also helps to visualize yourself in the speaking situation. Make it a positive visualization. Imagine yourself standing in front of the room. Picture individuals sitting in the audience, listening attentively. See yourself taking questions, answering them clearly and concisely. Hear the applause as you conclude. Visualization is an important part of your mental preparation. It helps you to reduce the effect of "stage fright." If you visualize your presentation in detail, you will feel some of the fear and nervousness which accompany public speaking. This may not make the fear and nervousness go away, but you will become accustomed to those feelings, and they will not disrupt your talk.

And now for something *really* scary ...

Two of the most frightening and, at the same time, most useful rehearsal tools are the *tape recorder* and the *video camera*. Your friends may give you constructive criticism with at least a little bit of sugar coating. The tape recorder and the video camera are cold, emotionless, and mostly honest in telling you how you did. Keep in mind that your voice might actually sound better live than it does coming from a tiny speaker. Still, the first time you hear or see yourself giving a presentation on tape you may feel a little intimidated.

Don't panic or give up! Do exactly what we suggested you ask your evaluators to do. Follow the three-step plan for evaluation. First, look for the things you did well, and take a moment to feel good about those things. Then, identify one or two things to work on for next time. And finally, give yourself credit for the improvements you have made since you began working on your presentation skills. It's hard to believe when you are starting out, but after you have practiced on tape a few times you will see considerable improvement. You may even begin to like yourself as a speaker.

The key is to work through those first few frightening episodes and *keep on practicing.*

Conclusion

Athletes and musicians, among others, can testify to both the occasional drudgery and the incredible value of practice. If you want to become a better speaker, you must make the effort. The payoff is worth the time you put into becoming a better speaker.

Some key messages from this chapter

- *Practice your talk aloud, not just "in your head."*
- *Be certain to stay within your time allotment.*
- *Get constructive feedback from your colleagues.*

Exercises

1 Practice your presentation using a video camera or tape recorder. Then replay the tape and *constructively* evaluate your performance. Remember to give yourself credit for the things you do well.
2 Ask a colleague or mentor to evaluate your next practice or presentation. You may provide a copy of our "Speaker Evaluation Guidelines and Checklist," or you may wish to point out specific skills you wish to improve.

Box 4.1 on next page

Box 4.1 Speaker evaluation guidelines and checklist

Guidelines for evaluating another speaker

- **First, highlight what the speaker did well.** Positive feedback is important. Reward is more effective than punishment; the carrot works better than the stick.
- **Suggest *one or two* ways the speaker may improve.** It's more useful to work on *one or two* things at a time than to try to fix everything at once.
- **Conclude by emphasizing something the speaker did especially well.** This may be something the speaker has genuinely done well, or it may be an area where the speaker has made great improvement.

Here are some *specific* things to look for when evaluating a speaker:

- Could you recognize and summarize in a sentence or two what the speaker's intended message was?
- Was the talk targeted to the level of the audience?
- Was the talk well organized?
- Did the visual aids clearly support the speaker's message?
- Did the speaker make good eye contact with the audience?
- Did the speaker speak clearly and loudly enough? Did the speaker use vocal variety?
- Did the speaker choose appropriate and effective words to convey the message?
- Did the speaker make effective use of gestures or other body language?
- Did the speaker convey enthusiasm for the subject?

Part II

Delivery

This section of the book deals with the actual delivery of your talk. Once you have gone through the preparation steps outlined in Part I, these aspects of your presentation will be far less intimidating. Careful and thorough preparation will give you confidence, and that confidence will spread throughout the "mechanical" aspects of your speech.

First, this confidence can help you to take control of the speaking situation. In Chapter 5 we discuss the responsibilities which fall to you when you agree to speak. When you accept and carry out these responsibilities you are *in control*.

Next, we examine voice and language, the most basic components of a speech. You can use volume, pacing, pitch, and other vocal qualities to convey your message most effectively. Word choice is especially important in technical presentations, and it must be appropriate to your specific audience. In addition, since much of science is discussed in English, and many scientists are not native English speakers, there are language issues which both native and non-native speakers must take into account.

In Chapter 7 we look at nonverbal communication: body language and facial expression. If these are consistent with your spoken words, your message is supported; if you exhibit fear and uncertainty, your listeners will be uncertain about your words as well. In this chapter we will discuss ways in which you can align your nonverbal signals with the story you want to tell.

Your job isn't finished until the questions have been answered. Question-and-answer sessions bring the fear of the unknown, but they also offer you some excellent opportunities. In Chapter 8 we consider how to make the most of the Q & A period.

Chapter 5

Take control of the situation

As the speaker, you must take charge of the speaking situation. This is no time to be tentative. If you appear to be comfortable and in control your audience will become comfortable too. In order to take control of your speaking event there are things you should do *before* you start talking, things you should do at the *beginning* of your talk, and things you should do *throughout* your presentation. In this chapter we will discuss each of these areas in detail. First, here is a quick overview.

1 Before the talk begins:
   - Make sure the room is set up properly
   - Take a few minutes to talk to your host and the early arrivals
   - Take a few minutes to get yourself mentally prepared
   - Have your opening sentences firmly in mind

2 At the *outset* of your talk, there are some more ways to maintain your control:
   - Be sure you are properly introduced
   - Let your listeners know what to expect
   - Let your listeners know what is expected of them

3 *Throughout* your talk, there are several other responsibilities which you must fulfill:
   - Display a positive, enthusiastic attitude
   - Connect with audience members using good eye contact and pauses
   - Stay within your time limit
   - Give a strong ending, then stop talking

Before you start talking

It pays to be an early bird. Arrive at least 30 minutes before your presentation. Stand in front of the room and survey your situation. Walk around the stage, looking over the seats, imagining the people who will soon be there. Survey your domain until you feel as if you own it.

Check the room set-up

Make sure that all of the audiovisual equipment works. Who controls the slide projector, and how? Project your slides and check the focus. Try out the microphone to ensure that it works and that you know how to operate it. Test your video or computer equipment thoroughly. Can everyone see the whole screen? Where are the controls for the lights? Will there be someone available in case of equipment or lighting problems? Do you have access to chalk, a pointer, or markers in case you need them? If you need a glass of water, now is the time to get it. Be comfortable in asking for anything you need – water, facial tissues, thermostat adjustments, opening a window for ventilation, closing a door to keep out noise. Remember, it's your show and you are taking charge.

To the extent possible, arrange the room to suit your needs – make it your own. Do everything you can to make yourself feel comfortable on-stage.

Talk to the people who arrive early

Do all of the room set-up far enough in advance so that you have time to chat with those who arrive early for your presentation. This will be your first opportunity to connect with your audience. It's your chance to ask more questions, to gather even more information about your listeners. What is this person's background and interest in your topic? What caused this person to come and hear you – what are the expectations? If you show an interest in your listeners, you will start the talk with some people already on your side, and you will feel less intimidated since your audience will be less of an unknown quantity.

Take a few moments for mental preparation and relaxation

The moments just prior to your talk can be the most terrifying. If you have found successful ways of dealing with stress in your life, try applying them to speaking situations. If you haven't, try one or more of these methods:

- Take a deep breath, then exhale in a slow, controlled manner. Repeat as needed; with each breath you will feel more calm. Exhale slowly – otherwise you will hyperventilate and faint!
- Some speakers like to dissipate nervous energy in physical ways, such as stretching or exercising, prior to their presentations. In the moments before you begin speaking you can do isometric exercises quite unobtrusively – tense and relax your leg muscles, or press your palms together.
- Repeat a mantra, a phrase or sentence which is meaningful, familiar, and reassuring. Dorothy Sarnoff, author of *Never Be Nervous Again*, recommends this one: "I'm glad I'm here, I'm glad you're here, I care about you, I know that I know." This focuses your attention on the audience (instead of on you) and puts your speaking situation in a very positive light. And it reaffirms to you that you are, in fact, an expert on your topic.

Have your opening sentences firmly in mind

Have your opening sentences memorized and thoroughly rehearsed. Once you get through the first few sentences your body naturally calms down – it can't go on producing adrenaline at high rates indefinitely. For most speakers, the first 30 seconds are the most stressful. Get through the first few sentences and you will find that you are on your way.

As you begin talking

Once you begin your talk you can make your audience feel comfortable. We're not talking about cushy chairs and refreshments. Your listeners will feel most comfortable if they know right away who you are and what you have planned for them. They also need to know when you wish to take questions.

Have we been introduced?

Prior to your talk, find out from your host who will be introducing you. Give this person enough information to introduce you properly. You can bring along a written introduction to be read if you wish. The introduction should tell the audience who you are and why you are there. It should let the audience know you are qualified to speak on the subject at hand.

Be prepared to introduce yourself in case you are not given an adequate introduction. What credentials entitle you to speak on this topic? You can do this without simply listing your degrees, patents, and publications. Here is an example:

> Today I want to tell you about some really exciting work we have done in building computer-based models of drug receptor sites. I first became interested in drug-receptor binding as a pharmacy student at the University of Wisconsin. In graduate school I synthesized analogs of drugs to study which conformations of drug molecules could activate receptors. For the past 17 years I have used computers to help in the task of drug design. Recently I have begun using a genetic algorithm to build receptor models, and that is what I want to tell you about today.

This five-sentence introduction establishes the speaker's educational background and years of experience, tells the audience that the speaker is enthusiastic about the work to be discussed, and leads directly into the specific topic of the talk.

Are you qualified? Many people with strong technical backgrounds feel that they are not expert enough. This is because the more we learn about a subject, the more we realize how little we really know. Relax! We all understand that no one can know *everything*. Chances are that you know a *great deal* more about your topic than anyone else in the room. And it is absolutely certain that no one else comes to this subject with the same background, experience, attitudes, and opinions as you. If you find yourself facing an audience which includes the world's leading authority on the subject, acknowledge his or her expertise and then tell your story to your assembled audience. Be proud that the world's expert took time to come and hear what you have to say. Even that expert doesn't know everything. You bring a new perspective and a new set of experiences, and that other expert may be the one who can best appreciate your message.

What can they expect from you?

Right up front, lay out your plan for the session. Introduce your listeners to your key message (which we identified in Chapter 1) as soon as possible. As we discussed in Chapter 2 (organization of your talk), the introduction should put your topic into perspective, and it should let people know the scope of the material you plan to cover. You probably can't do justice to a subject such as "immunology" in a 20-minute talk. What aspect of immunology do you plan to discuss?

Tell them what your time-frame is. If you have planned to talk for an hour, and half of your audience has to leave for another meeting or class in 30 minutes, it's better to find this out right away so you have time to adjust.

What do you expect from them?

In Chapter 8 we will discuss question-and-answer sessions in detail, but here we will point out that you are entitled to tell your listeners the rules for Q & A right up front. As the speaker, you get to make up the rules. If you fail to do so, you will have to play by the audience's rules, even if you don't know what they are. Do you want to take questions as you go, or do you want to avoid interruption and handle all questions at the end? There are pros and cons to each approach. You must decide which way you prefer to do it, and it is up to you to tell the listeners what you want.

Throughout your presentation

Attitude

One important component of taking control is an intangible: attitude. Be yourself. Look and behave as if you belong in front of the room. Act as if you are happy to be there. Practice and experience will help you achieve this. Remember that you have accepted a responsibility. Make yourself comfortable in this role. You are there to lead, inform, persuade, teach, entertain.

Keep in mind that the audience *wants* you to succeed. Even if they ask a few tough questions they do *not* want you to fail in your mission – that would be unpleasant for them as well as for you. Jimmy Stewart attributed his success as an actor to the attitude that you *treat the audience as your partners*. Ultimately, both the speaker and the listeners want a successful outcome, and neither can achieve it without the other. It really is a partnership

If you exhibit nervousness and fear, this makes your listeners feel uncomfortable. Unfortunately, this starts a downward spiral. You sense the audience's discomfort, and it makes you more uncomfortable. If you feel nervous, remind yourself: "I feel nervous because I am excited about this opportunity to share what I know with others. I am here because I have something to give to *these people*." By keying on your excitement to share with others, you put the focus on your message and your audience instead of yourself, and this will minimize the amount of nervousness which comes through to the audience. There is a very fine line between nervousness and excitement; one makes your listeners uncomfortable, while the other inspires them. Amazingly, your attitude and your focus can channel the energy to the "excitement" side of that line.

Make eye contact

Where are your eyes looking when you are speaking? There are many places where they should *not* be focused. Don't be glued to your notes or script. Don't spend your time looking at a screen or board, talking to your visual aids. Don't gaze down at the floor while you talk. Don't talk to the back wall or the ceiling. And don't stare up into your brain looking for your next thought.

As you speak, practice looking at individuals in your audience. When you look people in the eye, they have a tendency to trust you. If you seem to be avoiding eye contact they may feel that you are hiding something from them. Perhaps you are trying to hide your fear of public speaking, but they may subconsciously suspect that what you are hiding is connected with your message. Good eye contact is an important reinforcement for your spoken word. It says that you are sincere about your subject matter.

It may be difficult at first to get into the habit of making eye contact with your listeners, but it really is an important skill to master. When you make eye contact with your audience you convey sincerity. You involve the listeners more directly. And you once again help control your anxiety by focusing on the audience instead of yourself. Don't make the mistake of talking only to the most senior person in the room – include as many people as possible.

The key is to practice delivering one complete thought to one pair of eyes; if you dart around the room too rapidly you will look frantic. Connect with a pair of eyes and deliver one complete thought. Pause, connect with another pair of eyes, deliver another complete thought. Pause again, connect with another pair of eyes, and deliver the next complete thought. If you need to look at notes, do so during the pause. When you first practice this skill it may look and feel mechanical, but it will quickly become smooth and natural for you.

The one thought–one person skill serves another important purpose. It provides visual punctuation, giving the listeners important cues about when each thought begins and ends. Once you become adept at doing this you will make it easier for your listeners to get your message.

The pause between sentences is important. It lets your listeners process what you just said, and it lets you prepare for your next sentence. Many speakers are uncomfortable with silence at first. They run sentences together, or fill the silence with "um" or "ahh" or other sounds. To you, the speaker, the pause may seem eternally long, but it will *not* seem that way to your listeners. They will not be consciously aware of it; you will seem thoughtful, and you will be better understood. Make a conscious effort to pause between sentences, and you will soon become very comfortable with those moments of silence.

Please don't make it difficult for your listeners to make eye contact with you. If you put 20 lines of text on the screen, people will be so busy reading that they can neither look at you nor listen to what you are saying. Even if you manage to look at them they will not be looking back.

When you learn to look at your listeners one at a time you will notice that you can read their facial expressions and body language. You will recognize when you have made yourself clear. You will see when people are puzzled and need further clarification. You will notice that people are interested in what you have to say, and that will contribute to your comfort level as a speaker. When you put the focus on your listeners instead of yourself, you are less self-conscious, less nervous, and more in control of your situation.

Watch the time

There is one more component to audience comfort: watch your time limit. Even if your audience has been with you all the way, once you go past the time limit your listeners' minds rapidly move in other directions and their comfort level dives. As we discussed in Chapter 2, if you find that you must cut short your presentation, cut out details. Do *not* shorten or skip your conclusion. The conclusion should be the part of the talk which clarifies and emphasizes the key message. It's the one part of the presentation which should not be sacrificed or rushed.

Give a strong ending, then stop talking

Work on crafting a strong conclusion for your presentation. Just as you may wish to memorize the first few sentences of your talk, you may want to memorize the final sentence or two. Make sure your key message is reinforced. If you want your listeners to do something or believe something or buy something, this is the place to *ask for what you want*. If you've done everything else right, and then your talk ends weakly, you will probably not get the response you are looking for. Too often, talks end with a feeble "Thank you" or "Are there any questions?" or "So, um, that's all . . ." The best way to let people know you are through talking is to give a strong concluding sentence which ties things up neatly, and then to stop talking. Look around the room. Smile at your listeners. The first time you try this it will seem to you as if there is an eternal silence, but it really isn't long before people realize you are finished talking, and they will applaud or begin to ask questions.

Conclusion

When you are the speaker you are thrust into the role of leader. It is important for you to accept this role and to carry it out with confidence. This can be done if you prepare thoroughly and meet the needs of the audience. Before you start, prepare the room and prepare mentally. At the outset of your talk, be sure your listeners know who you are and what your expectations are. Throughout your talk, display enthusiasm and give one-thought-to-one-person eye contact.

Some key messages from this chapter

- *Before your talk: check the room set-up, check your visual aids, and take a few moments to mentally prepare yourself.*
- *At the outset of your talk: let your listeners know what to expect from you, and let them know what you expect from them.*
- *During your talk: display a positive, enthusiastic attitude, stay within your time limit, and give a strong ending.*
- *Make good eye contact with your listeners: deliver one complete thought to one pair of eyes, pause between sentences, then deliver the next complete thought to another pair of eyes.*

Exercise

This eye contact exercise is best done with a group of three to six people. At a pinch you can do it alone, speaking to photographs of people on your wall, or you can even practice on a small audience of pets or teddy bears.

Put together a two-minute talk about a subject which is very familiar to you. The goal is to have several sentences which you can say without notes and without having to think about content as you go along. You should be able to focus on delivering sentences while maintaining good eye contact.

Now look directly into the eyes of one person. Look until you can tell the color of the person's eyes. Give your first sentence while maintaining eye contact with this person. Complete the entire sentence before breaking eye contact. *Pause.* Get your next sentence in mind and make eye contact with another person. Be sure you have established eye contact before you start speaking. Continue this sequence (eye contact, complete sentence, pause) until you have delivered all of your sentences. Initially you may wish simply to go left-to-right so that you don't have to think about who to make eye contact with next. Don't be concerned if the process seems mechanical at first. Eventually you will be able to make your eye contact all around the room without having it look contrived.

Chapter 6

Voice and language

Perhaps you assume that your voice is something you are born with, and it can't be changed. Perhaps you take your voice for granted. But just as you can strengthen your biceps with exercise, you can improve your speaking voice with practice. Volume, pacing, and vocal variety are components which you can develop. Your choice of words is equally important in developing your speaking style. The language you use will determine whether you communicate or confuse. Later in this chapter we discuss the particular problems facing speakers who are using a language other than their native language, since this is a common situation in most scientific fields and technology-oriented careers today.

Voice

Your voice is the vehicle which conveys your words to the listener. If you speak in a flat monotone you take your listeners for a ride in a beat-up old car. With attention to volume, pace, and pitch, you can treat them to a trip in a zippy sports car – much more exciting. But don't make it a hair-raising, pedal-to-the floor ride in a racing car!

Volume

It's obvious: if you are not heard, you will fail as a speaker. If you are a quiet person, if you tend to be shy, if you are usually reluctant to speak up in conversations, you must recognize public speaking as a unique situation in which your usual style will not succeed. When you accept the responsibility of giving a presentation, you owe it to your listeners to make yourself heard. Accept the fact that you will have to put on a voice which sounds much too loud to you. Remember, your listeners are not inside your head, and some of them will be sitting in the last row of seats. Practice speaking in an auditorium, a large room, or outdoors. Imagine that the microphone has failed, and you have to speak loudly enough for everyone to hear. Become accustomed to the sound of your own loud voice. Finally, when you practice your presentation, ask someone to sit in the last row and check your volume for you.

Take advantage of the whole range of volume available to you. Suddenly lowering your voice to a near-whisper can make your listeners more attentive. Shouting clearly adds emphasis (provided you are not shouting all the time). Extremes of volume are very effective, but they should not be overused. Most of the time you can use more subtle variations in the middle regions of your volume range to keep your listeners interested and attentive.

If you are offered a microphone, please use it. Too many speakers (especially men!) act as though they have been insulted. A microphone? Do I look like a guy who needs amplification? "Can everybody hear me?" he shouts. No one in the audience speaks up – he's shouting, so of course they hear him. And those who can't hear will have missed the question. The speaker starts out talking loudly enough, but two minutes into the talk he reverts to his normal speaking voice. It isn't as though he is completely inaudible – it's just that the listeners must strain a little to hear. Don't make them work so hard. As a communicator you want to make it as easy as possible for people to get your message. The microphone makes it easier for your audience, and it lets you speak more naturally. You don't have to strain your voice. You can use the whole range of your vocal capabilities.

There are many kinds of microphones. Best are the wireless models which clip on. These keep your hands free and let you move anywhere in the room. Check before your presentation to be sure the batteries are working. If you will be using a microphone with a cord, practice with it so that you don't trip over it or knock your overheads onto the floor with the cord. Before you start talking, make sure you have enough cord to move around. When you must use a hand-held microphone, keep it a fairly constant distance from your mouth. If it's too close the volume becomes too loud and words get distorted; if it's too far away you become inaudible. Worst of all are microphones attached to the lectern. Now your mobility is truly limited, and you can't even move your head very much without disturbing that mouth-to-microphone distance.

Pacing

Speed is another vocal variable which we can control. We can think much faster than we can speak, so the most common problem speakers face is a tendency to talk too rapidly. Keep in mind that you already know your topic, so you can move through it quite quickly, but most of your listeners are less familiar than you. They need just a little more time to hear, process, and assimilate the information you are giving them. When we talk too rapidly it is easy to slur a syllable, or to skip a word or even a whole thought. One way to learn to slow down is to practice enunciating each syllable distinctly. If you find yourself rushing or sliding over some words, try *exaggerating* the enunciation, as though you are speaking over a noisy telephone line.

Another important pacing tool is the use of the pause. Like changing your volume, inserting a pause lends emphasis to what you have just said. It gives the listener time to process what you have just said, rather than having to hurry on to the next string of thoughts. Be sure to pause after you have made an important point, or you risk the possibility that some listeners will miss it.

Pauses seem to last forever when you are standing in the front of the room. Do the tape recorder experiment. Try speaking a few sentences using pauses. Note how long the pauses seem when you are speaking. Then listen to the tape – you will see that the pauses aren't so long after all. In fact, they can help to make your message easier to understand.

Many speakers are *terribly* uncomfortable with pauses. So uncomfortable, in fact, that they fill those pauses with noises such as *um, er, ah*. These sounds are quite distracting to the listener. Why do we use them? Picture yourself in a lively conversation with a large group of people. In that situation, if you pause, someone else jumps in and starts talking. Under those circumstances, a filler noise like *ahhhh* serves to hold your place, so that no one interrupts you. But if we let this habit (which is rooted in a fear of interruption) carry over to our public speaking style, it becomes a hindrance. When you are giving a presentation you will *not* be interrupted. You have the floor. You can cast aside that fear-based habit. You can make a point, then pause and watch it sink in. Try it. Make an important point, then pause and watch people in your audience.

You can literally *see* facial expressions change as the light bulbs go on. It's an exhilarating experience! Once you stand in front of an audience and wield the power of the pause you will feel liberated.

Closely related to those pause-filling sounds are "start-up" words. Some speakers start almost every sentence with words such as "So . . ." or "Okay." Why does a speaker begin his talk by saying "So, uh, today I want to tell you about . . ."? The "start-up" words are there to make sure the speaker has the listeners' attention before giving the message. Again, this may be a useful tool in a group conversation, but it serves *no* good purpose in an oral presentation. You, the speaker, are already the center of attention. Check the tape to see if you are unconsciously committing this error.

Pausing after a sentence serves several other purposes. It allows you to prepare mentally for your next thought. This helps to make your presentation smoother. The listeners won't mind if you pause to collect your thoughts – they will be using the time to assimilate your previous thoughts. The pause gives you the opportunity to continue making eye contact with your listeners. And as you make eye contact you will be able to gauge how well you are communicating with your audience. If people look puzzled, you can clarify your last point, or ask if there are questions. If people look bored, you may need to pick up the pace or increase your energy level.

Finally, pausing makes it easier for you to breathe properly. Under stress, we sometimes resort to rapid, shallow breathing. This can make your words and sentences sound choppy, and it limits the effectiveness of your voice. If you pause and take a deep breath before you start a sentence, you will speak more smoothly and you will be able to enunciate more clearly. There will be a simultaneous calming effect, since slow deep breaths help you relax.

Vocal variety

Chocolate ice cream is delicious, but if that were your whole diet for a week you would surely tire of it. If you use the same volume throughout your talk your listeners will tire of it as well. The words "monotone" and "monotonous" are *very* closely related. Give your presentation some variety. Changing your volume within a sentence gives your listeners important clues about what you want them to get. This is one of the primary advantages that your oral presentation has over your written work. (If I were *saying* that last sentence instead of writing it I would use changes in volume to emphasize the words "advantages," "oral," and "written.")

Be particularly careful not to let the ends of your sentences fade away. Check your tape recordings, or ask your evaluators to look for this common problem. The end of the sentence is often the most important part. If you simply increase the pitch and volume at the end of most sentences you can make a substantial difference. Try ending your sentences "up" (slightly higher pitch and volume). You will sound more positive, more authoritative, and more enthusiastic. But take care that you don't finish sentences with higher pitch and *less* volume – this makes you sound tentative or questioning.

Volume and pacing are just the beginnings of vocal variety. Pitch is important in conveying emotion and feeling. Lower pitch may carry a sense of calmness and logic, while higher pitch connotes more intense emotion. This doesn't mean that men always sound calmer and more logical than women. A deep-voiced man speaking at the high end of his pitch range may sound stressed and fearful; a woman with a high-pitched voice can sound most serious when using the low end of her range. The key is to exercise some of your range and to use it to reinforce your message. Are you excited about your topic? Raise your pitch a little! Do you need to be authoritative on a particular point? Dial down the pitch. But be careful. There is a natural tendency to lower the *volume* when you lower the pitch, and this may not be what you want.

Your voice is capable of conveying many positive qualities: confidence, friendliness, sincerity, enthusiasm. These qualities are more difficult to analyze than volume, speed, and pitch. While they receive expression in your voice, they originate in your mind. Confidence comes from knowing that you know your subject and from practice. Sincerity comes from sincerely wanting to share your message with your listeners. Enthusiasm is based on your feelings toward your topic. It's sometimes hard for logic-oriented technical people to accept (because we don't understand exactly how it works), but if you consciously consider that you do, indeed, want to share your knowledge with your audience, sincerity *is conveyed* in your voice. If you are excited about your subject and you decide not to suppress your enthusiasm, then your enthusiasm finds expression in combinations of volume, speed, pitch, and perhaps other vocal qualities.

Vocal variety is one of the best ways to prevent boredom in your listeners. You can use your voice to create expectation, so that people can't wait to hear the rest of the story. Variety enables you to accentuate the main points of your talk. Most importantly, it lets you insert some drama and life into your presentation, and this will make it an exciting and memorable experience for your audience.

Language

Our discussion of language will cover several important topics: our choice of words, proper pronunciation of words, issues faced by non-native English speakers when speaking in English, and issues which native English speakers must be aware of when the audience includes non-native English speakers.

Choice of words

Whether you are speaking to a junior high science class or a room full of doctors, clear and simple language is most effective. Certainly you can use a different vocabulary with the latter group, but don't choose complex words when simpler ones are available. The word "pedantic" describes the vain or ostentatious display of learning. Make sure you are not using big words simply to impress people. Choose the words which give clearest expression to your message.

Jargon is the two-edged sword of communication. Jargon exists because it is useful in everyday work. It saves time in writing and in conversing with colleagues. It's faster to say "DNA" than to say "deoxyribonucleic acid." But in technical presentations, jargon presents some hazards. First, listeners who are not familiar with a term must spend some time trying to infer what you mean, and this is time when they cannot pay full attention to your message. More seriously, these listeners may feel that you are slighting or excluding them, and they may become indifferent or even hostile to your message.

The most educated listeners will not have the same experiences and background that you have. They cannot know all the abbreviations and terminology you know. And even if they have heard of a Dieckmann condensation before, you do no harm by recapping it briefly for them. They will each think you are doing it for the benefit of someone else, and they will feel better about themselves for already knowing.

Your presentation will be much more lively and understandable if you use illustrative language. Roger Ailes, in *You Are the Message*, suggests using analogies from other fields to enliven your material and help the audience remember your key points. When you liken gel electrophoresis to animals of different sizes running through a dense forest, you paint a vivid mental picture, and you make your explanation much more memorable. You make it easy to see why large proteins move more slowly than smaller ones. Analogy can be a powerful tool in helping people to grasp abstract or difficult concepts.

Whenever possible, use *positive* language rather than negative. People respond much better to a positive message. If you are comparing your method (or product or result) with someone else's, it is much more convincing to talk in term of the *advantages* of yours than to harp on the *disadvantages* of theirs.

By the same token, remove *negative* language from your talk. Suppose you want to get an audience to accept your point of view. When you start your talk by saying "I will try to convince you . . ." you bring along the negative implication "but I might not." You are already making your excuses for failure. How can you convert this to a positive? When you say "I will show you why I believe . . ." you tell the audience in positive terms what you *will* be doing. If they cannot be convinced, it may be for reasons which have nothing to do with your presentation.

Double negatives tend to confuse listeners. "The failure to detect X-rays could not be taken to indicate that no fusion occurred" is a little difficult, since "failure," "not," and "no" are all negative. "We did not detect X-rays, but fusion may still have occurred" is probably clearer.

Finally, it is important (and also a little bit tricky) to use *precise* language. Cite a specific example rather than waving your hand and saying "et cetera" or "whatever." Naming a specific type of experiment or a specific laboratory will let your listeners know that the information is reliable. "Echinacea helps fight infection by boosting immunity" is less convincing than the statement "Echinacea helps fight colds by increasing the number of phagocytes, the white blood cells which ingest and destroy bacteria."

Watch out for expressions such as "They say that. . . ." Who says? Is this information coming from the National Academy of Science or from the Fruit Punch Advisory Council or from Aunt Helen? When you are specific about your source of information you give yourself credibility. But do this only to back up the main points. If you document every sentence, you'll footnote your talk into a mind-numbing bibliography.

Be especially careful when using statistics. These are *very* specific, but they can also be very hard to interpret. The state of New Hampshire has 5,013,000 acres of forest. Is this vast? Or is this just a small portion of the state? It may be more meaningful to tell the audience that 87 percent of New Hampshire's land area is forested. It might have an even greater impact to say that if your body were New Hampshire you would be covered with trees except for your head.

Pronunciation

Pronunciation is to the spoken word as spelling is to the written word. Many writers have wished that points would not be taken off for spelling mistakes, but in reality a spelling error will always be counted against you by some readers. Similarly, some listeners will take mispronunciation as a clue that you might not know what you are talking about. Don't fret about words which clearly have two accepted pronunciations – we don't mind that the word "methyl" is pronounced "meth' ill" by US-trained chemists and "mee' thile" by the British. But do take the trouble to check any word that you aren't 100 percent sure of. Use a dictionary, or, for technical terms, ask a colleague or two.

Pay careful attention to the articulation of your words. Use your tongue, teeth, palate, and lips so that each word is enunciated. Be especially careful to pronounce final consonants. For instance, be sure that "and" doesn't come out sounding like "an."

Back to Babel

The Book of Genesis talks about the importance of language in communication. The people of the world had only one language, and they built a tower which was to reach the sky. God's comment: "They speak one language. Soon they will be able to do anything they want!" Today scientists collaborate across national and continental barriers; companies are doing all they can to participate in global markets. If you can overcome language barriers you can accomplish almost anything.

Much of the world's technical communication is carried out in the English language. Most international scientific conferences, regardless of location, adopt English as the official language for the meeting. In the United States about 50 percent of Ph.D. degrees in the natural and physical sciences are earned by people for whom English is a second language. This raises important communication issues both for the English-as-second-language group and for native English speakers.

Language issues: when you are not speaking your native language

There are several things you can do to help yourself and your listeners if you must speak in English and it is not your native language.

1 Practice speaking frequently, and get some objective feedback about where you need to improve. We previously discussed the need to practice with an evaluator; in this situation, get a native English-speaking person to help you identify potential problems.
2 Practice reading aloud on a regular basis, both technical and non-technical materials. Tape-record your voice and listen to it. The ready availability of books on tape may help. Get the tape and listen to a portion of it. Then take the book and record yourself reading the same passage. Listen to yourself and compare your reading to that of a native English speaker.
3 Make sure you have included the important keywords in your visual aids. This way the main points will not be missed. But be careful not to put your whole talk onto your visual aids – if you do, your audience will read instead of listening.

Dr Lihong D'Angelo, a research scientist at the Coca-Cola Company, grew up speaking Chinese but has become highly skilled at giving scientific presentations in English. She reminds us that good scientific presentation in *any* language is an *acquired* ability. The key is to keep working on your skills, no matter what your situation is.

Language issues: when members of your audience are not native speakers of your language

Those of us who are native English speakers may feel that we have no language problems to worry about since we are rarely expected to speak anything other than English in technical fields. But keep in mind that your audience is likely to include a substantial number of people whose native language is *not* English. Your task in technical presentation is to communicate with *all* of your listeners. There are several steps you can take to help you connect with everyone in your audience.

1 Be especially careful about your choice of words. Look out for colloquial expressions. If you talk about an idea which is "out in left field," you are using a baseball-derived expression which may have no particular meaning to most of the world's population. Watch out, too, for references to old US television programs or literature. There are many people who don't know who Tom Sawyer is or how he got his fence whitewashed.
2 Be careful not to rush your speech. This is one more reason to make use of pauses (see pp. 87–1 on pacing). It is important to speak clearly and deliberately (without sounding patronizing).
3 Make sure you have included your keywords in your visual aids. This way the key points will not be missed. But be careful not to put your whole talk onto your visual aids.
4 When you are asked to repeat something your natural response may be to rephrase what you said; this can be confusing to a listener who has just partially translated what you said and now must start over. The first time you are asked to repeat something it's a good idea just to repeat it. If the listener still has difficulty then you may consider other ways to say what you mean.
5 When you are asked a question take the time to listen to the whole question. Resist the urge to help someone struggling with English by putting words into his mouth. Repeat the question to make sure you understand it.
6 Consider learning another language. It teaches you a great deal about your own language, and it attunes you to the importance of language issues.

Conclusion

As you practice, exercise your voice's range of volume, pitch, and speed. Look carefully at your choice of words, and be particularly aware of language issues, whether you have spoken English all your life or only for the last ten months. When you are in control of your voice and language you will be able to do anything you want.

Some key messages from this chapter

- *Vary the volume, speed, and pitch of your voice to emphasize your important points.*
- *Choose clear, straightforward language to convey your message.*
- *Watch for unnecessary jargon and slang terms which may not be familiar to all of your listeners.*

Exercises

Select a page from a textbook and record your voice as you read the page aloud. Listen to the recording. Did you vary your volume and pitch? Was the pace too fast or too monotonous?

Record the page again, paying attention to volume, pitch, and pace. Did your vocal variety improve? Listen again, paying attention to clarity of your pronunciation. Are the ends of your sentences strong and clear?

Look at the page one more time. If you were presenting this material orally what words would you change? How would you improve the clarity of the message?

Chapter 7

Body language and gestures

Your audience forms an impression of you before you open your mouth. Once you start talking your body language can support and reinforce what you are saying, or it can distract your listeners and detract from your message. What do you do with your hands? Where and how do you stand? Even the expression on your face can enhance your presentation. *You* are a visual aid!

First impressions

What is their first impression of you? Unless you emerge, speaking, from a cloud of smoke, your audience will form a first impression of you based on what they *see* rather than what they *hear*. And emerging from a cloud of smoke would, in its own way, make a visual first impression.

Whether it's fair or not, your listeners will have instant opinions about you before you say a word. Those opinions will be based, to some extent, on your clothing and grooming. This goes against the grain of many scientists and technical people. We want to be judged on the merits of our work. Perhaps it seems that using wardrobe and a haircut to impress listeners is cheating. At the other end of the spectrum there are numerous "dress for success" books which seem to suggest that you can craft a credible image based on appearance alone. Do you assert your independence, wear a T-shirt and jeans, and risk some portion of your credibility or impact? Do you cave in to convention and don the serious dark-blue suit? Or do you search for some middle ground?

To some extent, your choice depends on the event and the audience. Speaking to a group of engineers may not require the same dress code as speaking to a room full of corporate vice-presidents.

The atmosphere in a small company may be much less formal than that of a huge corporation. But dressing up tells your audience that you view your presentation to them as an important and special occasion. It shows that you are serious about your work. And it can boost your self-image and confidence. Once you are a more self-assured speaker you might not need the designer suit. If you observe speakers that impress you, though, you will find that they are almost invariably well groomed, with clean, pressed clothing.

The importance of nonverbal communication

When we talk with others we use nonverbal as well as verbal communication. Our face, hands, body postures and how we use the space around us convey impressions, and these are often emotional feelings rather than intellectual ideas. They can convey sincerity, honesty, openness, and receptiveness. On the other hand, if a person's body language is inconsistent with his words the audience becomes suspicious about the words.

Body language includes stance, posture, gestures, and facial expression. All of these kinds of body language can enhance your spoken message. To a large extent your body language is a matter of personal style; there is no single "best way to do it." But there are some general guidelines which we can offer. You can decide how best to incorporate these into *your* personal style. Let's take a closer look at some of these elements.

Facial expression

What does your face say about you? Are you happy to be there? If not, consider Anna in the Rodgers and Hammerstein musical *The King and I*. Whenever she feels afraid, she whistles a happy tune, and no one ever knows she's afraid. Then she realizes that "whenever I fool the people I fear, I fool myself as well." You *do* want people to get your message, so at some level you *do* want to be there. Smile, so that they will know you want to share with them. When you do this you will find that people respond positively, and you will eventually realize that you are, indeed, happy to be there.

One of the ultimate goals of this book is to put some life into technical presentations. Let people *see* the enthusiasm you feel for your subject Show that you are excited about your topic. Let them see you smile, let them see your eyes light up when you talk about the things that are important and interesting to you. Enthusiasm is infectious, and your listeners will catch it from you.

You will notice a difference in how eagerly your audience greets you if you step up to the podium with a spring in your step and a smile on your face. You have signaled the audience that you just can't wait to tell them something. Your enthusiasm will put them in a positive and receptive frame of mind from the start. Refer back to the section on "Take a few moments for mental preparation and relaxation" in Chapter 5 and you will find advice on how to put yourself in the proper frame of mind.

Posture

Standing in front of an audience can be intimidating. Many speakers are not comfortable being the center of attention. There is a natural tendency to try to hide. This leads to poor postures such as leaning on a chair or table, sagging shoulders, ducking one's head down, gazing at the floor, and hiding behind the lectern.

Posture is especially important. Be sure your back is straight and your weight evenly supported on both legs. Walk with books on your head until you are straight and proud. Also try pushing the top of your head against an imaginary ceiling until you feel it against your head. Push your shoulders down and distribute your weight evenly on the balls of your feet. Release your grip on any nearby furnishings.

If you hide behind the lectern you communicate fear. Learn to stand out in the open. Let the audience *see* you. To the extent possible, step away from the lectern and *toward* your audience. Get closer to your listeners. By doing this you break down a symbolic barrier. Appearing closer to the audience lets them know that you really do want to share your message with them.

Facing your listeners and making good eye contact are important components of body language. In Chapter 3 we discussed the danger of using your visual aids as your speaking notes. The more time you spend looking at the screen, the more time your audience must look at the back of your head (which happens to be less expressive than your face). And in Chapter 5 we learned the importance of eye contact in connecting with each member of the audience. Showing your face, particularly on a one-to-one basis, lets them know you really want to communicate with them.

What to do with hands and arms

What do you do with your hands and arms while you talk? You want your audience to be interested in watching you, not annoyed by watching you. We are amused by Thomas Leech's catalog of things *not* to do:

- Do not grip immovable objects such as furniture or lectern.
- Do not clasp hands in fig leaf position (in front of you) or in military at-ease position (behind your back).
- Do not have them hanging at your side, tensed in "gunfighter" position.
- Do not occupy them with pointer-waving, or coin and key jingling.

We would add to this list:

- Do not keep them in your pockets.
- Do not play with your hair, jewelry, necktie, or microphone cord.

So, what *should* you be doing?

- Let your arms hang straight, relaxed, at your sides.
- When you are not using your pointer, pen, or chalk, put it down or hold it still. If it is a laser light pointer, turn it off when it is not being used.
- Use your hands as you would in ordinary conversation: point or punch for emphasis, for example (but *never* point *at* someone).
- Make your hand and arm movements *larger*. Tiny gestures are not very useful if you are in front of a large room.

Accomplishing the task of being more expressive may require overcoming your self-consciousness. Unglue your elbows from your sides. Play with exaggerated gestures, imagine that you can feel the wind under your armpits, and this will help free you to use hands and arms naturally. Yes, think of it as play. Exaggerate and clown around in practice. It really does help you to feel less inhibited. If possible, have yourself videotaped. While you are practicing making expansive gestures, which may seem exaggerated to you, talk about how you are making bigger gestures than you usually would. Then watch the film. You will probably be shocked at how natural the movements actually appear. When you see with your own eyes how much more interesting you look by using more movement, it will make it easier for you to change your style.

More ways to be interesting to watch!

Practice being expansive, with gestures from the waist up, keeping the palms open and friendly looking. Bring your arms comfortably down to your sides when not speaking. Work through any self-consciousness, make your whole body part of your gestures, and soon you'll find people commenting on how lively your presentations are. Bending your knees, standing on tiptoes, and waving your arms might feel odd to you, but movement conveys the message that you really are into your topic.

For a particularly effective use of the space around you try the "step, turn, balance your stance and, POW, deliver the punch line" technique. When using visual aids you should use some variation of this method. Walk to the visual, point at it, then turn, find a pair of eyes, and, deliver the message. If you observe accomplished speakers you will see that many of them use the technique of taking a few steps, *in silence*, and then stopping, turning to the audience and delivering a message. Since the audience will be hanging on that silence, as they wonder what you will say when you break the silence, you could use either a quiet voice or a booming voice when you finally speak, and either would be powerful.

Summary

Your audience uses both sight and sound to receive your message. Make sure your visual message (posture, gestures, and facial expression) is fully aligned with the words you wish to convey. Try using more of the space around you, with expansive arm movement and moving about your stage. Synergy describes the situation where, when you combine two separate components, you get a more-than-additive result. This is what happens when you add a strong nonverbal component to your spoken words. People *really* get your message.

Some key messages from this chapter

- *Your appearance makes a first impression before you begin to speak. Consider ways in which you can make this first impression a positive one.*
- *Let your facial expression show your enthusiasm for your topic and your interest in communicating with your audience.*
- *Hands and arms: avoid distracting behaviors; instead, employ them in large, expansive gestures, especially if you are speaking in a large room.*
- *Face your audience with erect posture, coming out from behind the lectern when possible.*

Exercise

This one really is a physical *exercise*. Practice giving your talk in as large a room as possible. Experiment with exaggerated gestures. Imagine that you are in a very large auditorium, and that you want the people in the back row to be able to see your hand and arm movements. Make use of your entire stage area, walking across the space as you speak (but not pacing nervously!), and walking toward your audience to emphasize a main point. Most importantly, smile from time to time so that the audience can see that you are happy to be there.

Chapter 8

Handling question-and-answer sessions

What questions will they ask? The fear of the unknown can make the question-and-answer session the most intimidating part of your presentation. After all, you have control over what you say in your talk, but you don't have control over what your listeners may say afterwards.

Look at the positive aspects, though. This is your opportunity to detect and clear up any misunderstandings about your talk. You get another opportunity to reinforce your key message. And your audience can be your source for fresh input and new ideas about your work, if you are willing to listen.

Tell everyone what the rules are

Decide in advance when you wish to take questions, then let your listeners know up front. It is entirely up to you to decide whether you want to take questions as you go along, or at the end of your presentation, or at specific points along the way. For example, you could say "After I give you the background to this problem, I'll stop for questions, and then I'll be glad to answer any further questions at the end of the talk." You may wish to set aside time for questions after you have completed one major point, before you move on to the next, especially if a clear understanding of the first point is required in order to comprehend the next one.

Some speakers invite the audience to ask questions at any time during the talk. This tells the audience that you really want them to understand your presentation, but it has a lot of potential for problems, too. Impromptu questions may disrupt the smooth flow of your presentation. Every audience has the person who wants to race ahead and ask questions about later parts of your talk. And sometimes an audience can take you down a sidetrack which can completely derail your planned presentation. If you decide to invite as-you-go questions, be prepared to work harder at staying on course! One method of taking questions as you go is to hand out note cards to everyone, and to appoint someone to collect audience questions during your talk. At the end of your talk, you inform them, you will answer as many of the "anonymous" questions as time allows.

David Peoples suggests that the end of your presentation may be the *worst* place to take questions. If you are trying to sell a product, or to convince an audience about an idea, you may not want your carefully crafted closing statement to be followed by an unpredictable question-and-answer session. He suggests that you handle any questions, *then* give your closing comments.

How to handle questions

The first rule in answering questions is to listen to the *whole* question before you begin answering. This sounds simple, but there is a natural tendency to start formulating your answer as soon as you *think* you know what is being asked. You may tune out the questioner and begin thinking about your answer, and you could end up missing the real issue.

The second rule is to repeat the question. This confirms that you understood the question correctly, and it is helpful to audience members who could not hear the question in the first place. This is especially important if you are using a microphone and the questioner is not. If you are unable to understand the question well enough to repeat it, ask your questioner to repeat or clarify the question. When you repeat the question you get the opportunity to restate it for further clarity. It gives you an extra moment to compose your thoughts. Finally, it offers you the chance to reframe a truly hostile question.

The third rule is to answer the question concisely and then stop talking. The asking of a question is not your cue to give another ten-minute speech. If you talk too long you risk getting into far more depth than anyone finds interesting (yes, the details interest you, but most people just want to understand the big picture). And you risk going far beyond your allotted time. Time and listener attention spans are limited resources which you must manage carefully. There is also the danger that you may spend all of your discussion time on a single question, depriving others who wish to ask questions.

In formulating your answer, keep in mind your key message and, to the extent possible, relate your answer to that message. This helps you to focus your answer, and it often gives you a good way to wrap up your reply rather than rambling on endlessly.

What about the dreaded question you can't answer? Don't bluff or pretend that you know. Chances are that *someone* in the audience does know the answer, and you will be caught in an embarrassing situation if someone catches you. It is perfectly permissible to say "I don't know the answer to that one." No one is expected to have all the answers. In some situations you may wish to tell the questioner that you will research the answer and get back to him or her later. In some situations there may be others in the audience who know the answer. If you suspect that someone present knows the answer, and you believe it is useful to do so, you can ask whether anyone has the answer. But be careful about taking the approach of calling on a specific person out of the blue – you may embarrass a listener if he or she doesn't know the answer or wasn't paying attention at that moment. Questions with only two or three possible answers may lend themselves to a simple polling of the audience: "How many of you think the result will be an increased mutation rate? How many think the rate will decrease?"

You can, and should, anticipate some of the questions which may be asked. In your practice sessions ask your evaluators to question you so that you can practice your question-and-answer skills. And if you get a question you can't answer, go home and look it up; the next time you talk about this topic someone else is likely to ask the same question, and there is no excuse for not knowing the answer the second time.

The question-and-answer period is one more reason to have simple, clear visual aids. Marginally relevant details can sidetrack your talk, inviting listeners to pursue questions about things away from your main point. If you list details of the buffer and pH conditions you used, you encourage someone to interrogate you about why you used that particular buffer ("We always use a different one in our lab!"), and you can get distracted from the *result* you wanted to talk about.

How to handle hostile questions and questioners

As we discussed earlier, it is best to think of your audience as your partners. Occasionally, though, you may encounter a truly hostile questioner. Stay calm. If the questioner is hostile and you stay calm, pleasant, and polite, the audience will see the contrast and will tend to be on your side. On the other hand, if *you* are perceived as arrogant or hostile the audience may turn against you and proceed to grill you mercilessly.

Start out by acknowledging the questioner (without necessarily agreeing with his or her point of view). A statement like, "You bring up a very important (or interesting) point," gives your questioner credit for contributing to the discussion, and allows you to proceed to give your viewpoint on the subject.

If a question is posed in such a way that you cannot possibly give an acceptable answer you may need to reframe the question. Sometimes these questions start something like this: "It is well known that . . . [insert a questionable premise here] . . . so how can you conclude that . . . [insert your key message here]." If you simply restate your point of view without addressing the questionable premise, you will make no headway. Instead, you must reject any faulty assumptions and, if necessary, restate the question in a way which you believe is fair and reasonable. Then you can proceed to answer it rationally. Here is an example:

> *Question:* Enzymes do their work in solution, not in crystals, so how can you conclude that an X-ray crystal structure tells you anything useful about the nature of a protein in solution?

> *Answer:* Protein crystals typically contain about 50 percent solvent, and in some cases it is possible to diffuse substrate into a protein crystal and observe product formation. Therefore it appears that protein crystals behave very much like proteins in solution.

Sales people handle customer concerns using the "feel–felt–found" technique, and you can sometimes employ a version of it to handle hostile questions. Here is how it goes: "I understand why you *feel* that way about my methodology. I *felt* some concerns about whether it would work or not myself in the beginning, but I carried out a series of rigorously controlled experiments and I *found* that the method is very robust." You begin by acknowledging the questioner's feelings (without agreeing or disagreeing). Then you validate their feelings by pointing out that others (perhaps even you) have shared those feelings at one time or another. Now you can present other information which may convince your questioner to consider another point of view.

Sometimes people just have to agree to disagree. The question-and-answer session is not an occasion where you are likely to change long-held opinions, so don't let it decay into bickering about things which cannot be resolved immediately. You may have to terminate such a fruitless line of discussion with a comment such as "I can see that we have different opinions on this question, and only further research will show which of us is closer to the truth. Let's move on to other questions."

Once in a while you will encounter the person who uses the question-and-answer session to stand up and give his own little presentation, without ever asking a question (or with a trivial question such as "Don't you agree?"). If no question has been asked, you are not obligated to formulate an answer or to agree or disagree. You can simply say "That's an interesting comment."

If listeners give you helpful suggestions or comments this does not qualify as hostile questioning! Too often speakers immediately begin arguing, or start searching for reasons to dismiss the listener's idea. Don't do that! The questions or comments you get may be telling you that parts of your talk were not presented clearly enough. This can help you to improve your next presentation, and it offers you the opportunity to improve the clarity of the present one. If you are certain that the audience is clear about your message and they still differ with you, listen. People who have different experiences and who have taken the time to listen to your story are often the best source of new perspectives and new ideas. At the very least, give them credit for bringing up a good point, and thank them for doing so. Not all of these suggestions will be Nobel Prize material, but many of them will help you identify the places where you need to do more work. Take it as a compliment that your work stimulated some discussion!

Think about your audience

Keep the question-and-answer session under control. When you begin to take questions look around the entire room. Make sure everyone gets a chance to ask questions, not just the pushy guy in the front row. The rest of your audience will become restless and resentful if one person monopolizes the question time.

Occasionally the question-and-answer session turns into a private discussion among just a few people who are part of an in-group. If you see this starting to happen there are two things you can do. First, when you answer a question be sure to talk to everyone, not just the questioner. Second, make an extra effort to take questions from other people. This is especially difficult to do if the questioner happens to be a person of power or rank, such as your boss, but it is important that you make the effort.

Watching the time during Q & A is as important as watching the time during your presentation. There are numerous stories of the salesperson who has made the sale, then keeps on selling until the customer gets irritated and changes his mind. Be mindful of each listener's time, and if you know that a particular question is going to require a lengthy answer, give a brief answer and offer to go into detail with that person later.

Conclusion

It certainly seems to many speakers as if the question-and-answer period may be the most frightening part of giving a presentation. Once again, it pays to have in mind a key message to keep your answers focused. Do everything you can to break down barriers between you and the audience. Don't hide behind a lectern; come out into the audience and take their questions. Remember that the audience members are your partners. In a large lecture hall it may be hard to hear a question from the twentieth row, so go out and meet them halfway. Then, when you have heard the question, repeat it so that everyone hears it. Keep your answer brief and to the point. If questioners want lengthy, in-depth discussions, encourage them to speak with you further after the presentation. View the question-and-answer session as your opportunity to clarify your message one more time and to learn from your listeners.

Some key messages from this chapter

- *Decide in advance when you want to handle audience questions, and let your listeners know what the rules are.*

- *Listen to the entire question before you begin to answer. Repeat the question to make sure you understand it and to ensure that all listeners have heard it.*
- *Keep your answer brief and to the point. Relate it to your key message.*
- *Keep your question-and-answer session under control. Watch the time. Make sure everyone has an opportunity to participate.*

Exercise

When you practice your presentation, enlist one or more colleagues to listen and to ask questions. Your practice will be especially effective if you can get them to ask some difficult questions. Ask them to note the following:

- Did the speaker listen to the entire question before answering?
- Did the speaker repeat the question before answering?
- Were the answers concise and consistent with the key message?
- Was the speaker honest when dealing with questions that he or she could not answer?
- Did the speaker remain calm when faced with hostile questions?

Part III

Special situations

When you take up public speaking you will encounter a number of situations which do not fall neatly into either "Preparation" or "Delivery." We have put some of these topics into their own section at the end of this book. You will see that the skills you learned in the first eight chapters continue to be useful.

Unexpected things happen. You may be asked to give a visiting VIP a brief description of your work on the spur of the moment. Something may go wrong in the middle of your presentation. In Chapter 9 we look at ways to deal with these intimidating situations.

Once you have written a paper or given a presentation you may be asked to modify it for another occasion. You don't necessarily have to repeat the entire preparation process, but there are some steps you should not skip over. Adapting material from one source or from one audience to another is the subject of Chapter 10.

Finally, there may be times when you are called on to organize a program involving several speakers. The things you learned in previous chapters will, with some modification, enable you to do this most successfully. In Chapter 11 we tell you how to arrange and run a smooth and coherent session.

Chapter 9

When the unexpected happens

Life doesn't always follow the script you had in mind. Sometimes you are faced with unexpected situations: someone important stops by and asks for an impromptu description of your work, or something goes wrong in the middle of your planned presentation. In this chapter we look at how to handle extemporaneous speaking opportunities, and we discuss what to do when calamity strikes your presentation. Throughout this chapter the key message is: stay calm!

Extemporaneous speaking

Your hard-won presentation skills can serve you well when it comes to extemporaneous speaking situations (or even in your everyday conversation). You may be asked to talk about your work much more often in spur-of-the-moment, one-on-one discussions than in formal presentations. Many of the principles we have already learned can be used in these situations.

When the extemporaneous situation strikes . . .

Stay calm. A thoughtful pause is much more palatable than a string of filler sounds (um, um, ah, so, . . .). Take that deep, slow breath.

The big fear in extemporaneous speaking is "What happens if I can't think of anything to say?" We talked previously about ways to handle fear, and one of the best is to place your focus on the listener and the message instead of on yourself.

Apply the same methods you used for a rehearsed presentation. First, target your talk. Who is your audience? It is often helpful to ask a question or two to find out who you are talking to, what they already know, and what they want to know from you.

If you have gotten accustomed to the idea of focusing on a key message you have taken a big step in the right direction for extemporaneous situations. Take a moment to identify your key message. If you only have a short time to talk, it will be essential to keep the scope of your message fairly narrow. Focus on your single key message, and build on that focus as you talk. Don't ramble on just to fill time. Once again, resist the urge to tell everything you know. Stay close to your key message, and when you have delivered that message stop talking.

Follow the same rules as before for visual aids. Use simple diagrams. Most of the time it is more effective to draw a simple schematic diagram than to laboriously draw in every detail or to go rummaging through your files to find just the perfect picture. If you are in a position to write on a board, keep it brief. Bullet points are a quick and easy way to summarize. You may wish to write down keywords for emphasis.

Extemporaneous speaking situations are usually far less formal than other types of presentations. You can use this to your advantage. Your talk can be much more conversational and interactive. As you talk, you can ask questions which involve the listeners, turning your monologue into a dialogue. This also lets you decide as you go along what level of explanation is appropriate for your listeners.

Can you practice for an extemporaneous talk?

Here, too, what works for formal presentations will work for you in these spontaneous situations – practice. Pick one of your favorite topics and talk about it off the top of your head for five minutes. Or imagine that the President of the United States stops by your place of work and you are asked to describe what you do for a living, with a three-minute time limit. Think about how you would do it. What would be the key message? What would be the main points you would want to make? How would you sum it all up?

With a little practice you will reach the point where you could, with five minutes preparation, deliver a 30-minute talk. Spend a minute formulating the key message, two minutes thinking through the main points, and two minutes writing up an outline. This is a great all-purpose speaking exercise. It forces you to talk without relying excessively on visual aids. It makes you focus on the really important points (you don't have time to dig into details). And it makes you work from fairly limited notes rather than a detailed script. It's the oratorical equivalent of pumping iron!

The job interview as an extemporaneous situation

At one time or another almost everyone goes through a job interview. This may seem to be the ultimate extemporaneous speaking situation – they can ask you anything about anything. But there are many things you can do to manage the event.

Know what your key message is. What are you selling? You are selling yourself, your skills, and your knowledge, of course. Be prepared and skilled at giving the three-minute summary of who you are and what you can do. Be ready to give a specific example to illustrate each point you want to make. If you want to emphasize your initiative in finding creative ways to solve problems, don't just say "I can find creative ways to solve problems." That sounds like an interview truism. Instead, tell of a specific situation in which you found a creative solution to a difficult problem. That story is much more likely to make a lasting impression on your listener.

Too often the first-time job seeker thinks of the interview as an inquisition, one in which every question must be answered correctly. In reality, the interview should be a *dialogue*. The interviewer wants to see if you will fit his or her needs, and the interviewee ideally wants to see if the interviewer's situation is appropriate for him or her. If you are the interviewee, be prepared to ask questions as well as to answer them. Turn the interview into a conversation in which each party wants to find out about the other. Some interviewers are uncomfortable (or not very good at) asking questions. If you ask questions you take some of the pressure off the interviewer, and you show that you are interested in the position you are interviewing for.

You also need to know the difference between open-ended questions and close-ended questions. A close-ended question is one such as "How long were you at your last job?" for which the answer can be one or two words. An open-ended question is one which opens the door for discussion, such as "What do you expect to accomplish in the next five years?" Open-ended questions offer you the opportunity to deliver those key messages you wanted to bring out. If you are getting nothing but close-ended questions you may need to find a way to work your key message into the answer.

If you have been invited for an interview, chances are good that someone has already decided that your technical skills are sufficient. The interview is the time for the prospective employer to judge your interpersonal skills. If you can answer the interviewer's questions, ask your questions, and deliver your key messages in the course of the interview, you will have demonstrated your excellent communication skills.

When crisis strikes

Your slides missed the plane. The projector bulb burns out. The computer crashes. The fire alarm goes off. Someone faints from the heat. People in the third row are talking loudly. What do you do when things go wrong?

Stay calm

The most important thing for you to do in any crisis situation is to remain calm. If the situation occurs during your presentation the audience's reaction will depend to a large extent on your reaction.

Plan ahead

Take steps to avoid crisis wherever possible. When you are traveling, keep your slides in your carry-on bag, and not in the suitcase that accidentally ends up in Bloomington, Illinois instead of Bloomington, Indiana. Check the audiovisual equipment before your talk, find out where the spare bulbs are, and find out who to contact in case of equipment failure.

If your visual aids are lost or damaged, or unusable because of equipment failure, you will simply have to make do with what you have available: blackboard, markers, or whatever else you can find. Use visual aids only where they are essential to your talk. Draw simple schematic diagrams. Remember, an oral presentation is usually not a place for details anyway. Keep your improvised visual aids as simple as possible.

Deal with the situation as directly as possible

When the problem can't be avoided, stay calm, and deal with it as directly as possible. If you are being distracted by loud talking in the hallway, many members of your audience are certainly being distracted too. You must take steps to handle the problem. This could include closing a door, asking someone in the room to close the door, or asking the people involved to please move elsewhere.

It is up to you to ask for what you need. You can close a door to keep out noise, open a window to get some air, or close the curtains to keep out distractions. You may have to ask audience members to hold questions until the question-and-answer session. If the audience gets completely out of hand, you may have to ask people for some quiet so you can talk.

If there has been a disruption (tornado drill, falling chandelier, or an audience member carried out on a stretcher, for example), acknowledge the event, then go on. In some situations you might use humor to re-focus your audience. After everyone returns from the tornado drill you could say "Now that the storm has blown over, let's return to . . ." In other situations humor would be ill-advised: "We all hope that Dr Smith wasn't seriously hurt. Now we must return our attention to . . ."

Conclusion

In all sorts of unexpected speaking situations the audience will stay with you if you remain calm and confident. Remember the basics: stick to your key message, focus on the needs of the audience, and keep your illustrations simple.

Some key messages from this chapter

- *Stay calm, no matter what happens.*
- *Stay focused on your key message.*
- *Plan ahead for those potential problems which you can antici-pate, such as audiovisual equipment failure.*

Exercise

Try the exercise suggested earlier in this chapter: pick a topic with which you are familiar; then, with five minutes of preparation, deliver a 30-minute talk. Spend a minute formulating the key message, two minutes thinking through the main points, and two minutes writing up an outline. Then give the talk!

Chapter 10

Adapting material from one situation to another

Last month you gave a 45-minute in-house presentation on your latest research findings, and now you have been invited to discuss your work in a 15-minute session at a national conference. Last year you wrote a 20-page report describing your company's competitive position in antibiotic production facilities, and now your boss wants you to prepare a ten-minute presentation for the planning committee. There is the temptation to invest less effort in planning for the new talk, since you have already put the material together. Must you start from scratch each time? No, but there are some things to watch out for when you adapt material from one situation to another.

What has changed?

What lessons did you learn from your previous presentation? Did the talk flow smoothly? Did the questions suggest that something was not explained well? Did your key message come across clearly? Did your conclusion reinforce that message? If you haven't already done so, perhaps you should solicit feedback from colleagues who were present for your previous presentation. Ask for suggestions as to how you can improve your talk.

It is especially important to analyze your new audience and their specific needs. This part of your preparation cannot be shortened the second time around. Even if it happens to be the *same* group of people you are speaking to, time has passed and their needs may have changed.

With your new audience (and perhaps new time constraints), you then must evaluate your key message. Is the old one still appropriate? Do you need to modify it? If your allotted time is substantially different you may need to narrow or broaden the scope of the material you are covering. If this is the case, how will your key message change?

Once you have identified your new audience, and your adapted key message, you have to decide whether the organization you used previously is still useful. If the emphasis of your message has changed (from how you made the discovery to how that discovery will be exploited, for example), you may need to change the organization of your material completely. On the other hand, if you are just extending your previous talk to cover a little bit more ground your previous approach may do nicely with minor modifications.

Adapting written material to an oral presentation

If you have gone to the trouble of writing a report, a paper, or a book, you may feel that you have already prepared your material. Still, there are several things you need to do in order to make your written work into a first-rate talk.

Naturally, you have to identify your audience and their needs. The audience for your talk may differ from the intended audience for your written work. Also, you have to decide whether you are presenting the entire contents of your written work, or some portion of it. Do you need to focus on a particular part of your paper? Do you want to change your emphasis? Once again you have to identify your key message. These steps are part of the preparation for any talk.

In addition, there are some specific things you need to watch for when adapting written material to an oral format.

Oral presentation must focus on the main points and downplay details. Written material is intended to be more permanent; in addition to results, you usually describe in detail how you arrived at those results. Technical papers often include a section on materials and methods, so that readers can judge for themselves whether the results are valid. The oral format has a different purpose: to communicate the high points, the results, the essence of the subject. Those who are really interested in the details will want to talk to you further or read your book or buy your product. This may be the reason you are giving the talk – to get people interested in the details or the product. But the talk is not the place to lay out all that detail. Even in a classroom lecture you would not read a table of data to your class – you would spend your lecture time discussing why that table of data is important, or the major trends in the data, or how the data are applied.

An oral presentation also offers you the opportunity to tell your story in a more personal way than you could in a technical paper. You can inject some of your own personality and illustrate the talk with some personal anecdotes to bring the presentation to life. Take advantage of this opportunity!

Pay particular attention to the use of graphics from published material. You already went to a lot of trouble to make the graphs for your paper. Can you simply photograph or photocopy them to make your visual aids? Probably not. Look at (a) in Figure 10.1, a typical publication-quality graph. It is perfectly acceptable in print, but it will make an awful visual aid, even if enlarged The lines are too thin, the text is too small, and you won't be able to read the numbers on the axes. In (b), this graph has been adapted for use as a visual aid. Notice the changes. Titles and axis labels have been simplified and enlarged. The font has been changed to a sans-serif font (Helvetica), which usually projects better than serif fonts such as Times. The axes and data lines have been thickened, and the data points have been enlarged. The legend has been omitted.

Adapting a talk from one audience to another

Almost all technical work is interdisciplinary. This means that your work on new pesticides derived from plants may be of interest to entomologists, botanists, chemists, agricultural scientists, and environmentalists. You can't simply pull out the same set of slides for each of these audiences. Each group will demand a different emphasis. This is not to say that the entomologists are not interested in the chemistry or the environmental impact, but they will rightly want to hear more about the specific insects affected, whereas the audience of chemists may find that aspect far less interesting.

In our example, let us suppose you were formally trained as a chemist, and you have spent the past five years working on new pesticides derived from plants. It is entirely normal to be a little nervous when speaking to people outside your area of expertise. Are you qualified to speak to a group of entomologists or botanists? Would you be intimidated at the prospect of talking to a group of environmentalists? If you have been invited to speak, then someone

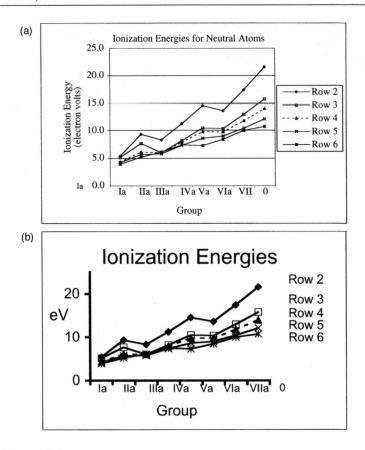

Figure 10.1

else has already determined that you are qualified – you know something that other people want to hear about. The group of botanists doesn't expect you to become an expert in botany before you arrive. They probably want to hear about what you are *doing* with a particular group of plants. Consider this: you will have an opportunity to talk with experts in botany, who may be able to point you toward other plants with similar activities which you were not aware of. Every challenge is an opportunity in disguise. As we pointed out in Chapter 8 (question-and-answer sessions), one of the major rewards for giving a talk is that you get the opportunity to learn and benefit from the experience of your listeners.

How do you approach a presentation to people with a very different background and expertise? First, find out all you can about your audience: their interests, their needs, their expectations. Don't waste time worrying about what you *don't* know. They want to hear about what you *do* know. Put special effort into your introductory material. Place your material into a frame of reference which is appropriate for your audience. Give sufficient background material so that they can appreciate your main points. Look for good analogies to help your listeners understand new concepts. And, as in any good talk, skip the unnecessary details in favor of the key results. In this example, even though you carried out deliciously clever experiments to determine the chirality of the naturally occurring pesticides, your environmentalist audience is much more interested in the fact that these compounds have existed in nature for millions of years. You probably need to concentrate on the fact that chemistry is being applied to the problems of discovering nature's stockpile of chemical weapons.

Adapting a long presentation to a shorter one

Can you squeeze your 40-minute talk into a 20-minute time slot by talking faster? By skipping every other sentence? We don't want to be in the audience when you do that experiment! Naturally, you need to do the same kinds of planning as before. How are the audience needs different in this situation? What is to be your key message? In particular, what changes will you need to make in order to fit your time limitations? Can you do this by reducing detail? Do you need to narrow the scope of your talk? Will this necessitate a major reorganization, or can you make do with minor modifications of your original outline?

Do you need to make new visual aids? There is a real temptation to recycle the old ones, since making new ones takes time. You need to be honest with yourself in looking at each visual aid and deciding if it fits your new situation. If the data have changed, you need to make a new visual aid. If you only need a part of the material on an existing visual aid, you should make a new one; the unused material on the old one could only serve as a distraction to your listeners, and it is likely to lead to questions that you may not have time to address. If an existing visual aid is not directly relevant to the new presentation, *leave it out*. This sounds obvious, but many speakers just load the carousel with the same old set of slides, then flash past the ones they aren't using. Once again, it is a distraction to the audience, and it is one which is easily avoided. Finally, if a new visual aid is required, take the time to make it. If your whole presentation is done with 35 mm slides, take the time to make another slide – don't disrupt the flow of your presentation by switching to an overhead and then back to slides.

Summary

When you adapt material from one situation to another, pay close attention to the steps which are critical for any talk:

* Identify your audience and their needs
* Identify your key message
* Make sure your organization is appropriate to your new situation
* Make sure your visual aids support your key message and are appropriate to your new audience

Do these things well, and your new talk will be a real success.

Some key messages from this chapter

* *When adapting material from a written format or from a previous talk, analyze your new audience. How does it differ from the previous audience? Does the key message need to be modified?*
* *When converting written materials to an oral presentation, focus on putting your talk into context for the audience and on the main points of your story. Stay away from details.*
* *When you have to shorten a talk, make a conscious decision about what material will be left out. Decide whether you need to narrow the scope of the material you will cover.*
* *When modifying a talk you have given before, check to see if your old visual aids contain extraneous information. If necessary, make new visual aids.*

Exercise

Look at the last presentation you gave.

1   Suppose that you had to cover this topic in one-half the time you used previously. How would you change your presentation? Would you narrow the scope of your talk? Would you cover the same material in less depth? How would you change your visual aids?

2   Suppose that you were asked to speak on this topic for twice as long as your previous presentation. What would you add? Would your key message be altered?

Adapting material: a checklist

-   In the first presentation, did I meet my goals and the audience's needs?
-   What did I do most successfully in the first presentation?
-   What do I most need to improve from the first presentation?
-   How is this audience different from the previous one? How are their needs different? Are my goals different?
-   How do I need to adapt my key message?
-   Is the original organization still appropriate?
-   Am I putting my message into a suitable context for this audience?
-   Am I focusing on the main points or getting bogged down in details?
-   Are my visual aids clear? Does each one directly support my new key message?
-   Have I adapted the scope of my talk to fit comfortably into the time available? Or am I trying to put too much material into too little time?

Chapter 11

Organizing a program with several speakers

There are several situations in which you may need to organize a program which includes several different speakers:

- You have been asked to organize and chair a session on semiconductor design as part of a national conference.
- You must coordinate a technical sales presentation which will involve presentations by you and three of your colleagues.
- You are asked to take charge of your department's weekly seminar program, which includes talks by department members as well as visiting speakers.

Let's look at some of the special challenges raised by these situations.

Coordinating the messages

If you are putting together a symposium or a group presentation it is important to come up with a unifying theme. What is the symposium all about? What is the goal of your group presentation? We start with our now-familiar process of identifying the key message or unifying theme. Who is the audience, and what are their needs? What are the goals of the presenters? The audience's background and needs may be fairly broad or highly specialized, depending on the situation. The national symposium on semiconductor design might bring together quite a diverse group of listeners and speakers. The theme might be "Recent Advances in Photomask Design and Production," which could attract listeners from several different disciplines. The technical sales presentation would undoubtedly have a sharp focus on the product or service being sold: "The Patagonia Corporation's combinatorial libraries offer the most diverse and convenient collection of chemical structures for your high-throughput bioassays," for example.

If you are organizing a weekly or monthly department seminar program it may not be necessary, or even desirable, to have such a common theme. You may need to have diversity in your program so that many different needs and interests can be met. It is often useful for such programs to include topics which are far outside the everyday interests of department members, just to bring in some variety and some fresh points of view.

Choosing the speakers

How many speakers do you need? Who will be your speakers? How much latitude do you have in choosing who will speak?

How many?

You have to decide how many speakers are appropriate. How much time is available? How much time will each one have to speak? Don't forget to allow time for discussion, coffee breaks, and meals when arranging longer programs. Audiences usually can't sit through four straight hours of non-stop talk.

Symposium program

Who are the authorities on the topic you have chosen? You may already know most of them if it happens to be your area of expertise. As you talk to each one, however, ask who else is doing exciting new work in this area. You may uncover good speakers you were not aware of. Similarly, if one of your world experts is too busy and turns you down, inquire about co-workers who might be qualified to come and speak. Don't give up too easily.

Technical sales program

When you are putting together a technical sales presentation you may have specific constraints: Dr Einstein has to be invited since he was the inventor, or you are required to include someone from research, someone from product development, and someone from marketing. Who, in each department, is skilled in oral presentation? Who is qualified to talk on the subject? Unfortunately, it's not always the skilled speaker who knows the subject best (that's why we wrote this book!). In such situations you may need to help your speakers with targeting, organizing, and visual aids. It will also be your job to coordinate among the different speakers to make sure that the key message is delivered consistently and clearly, to make sure that all aspects of the subject are covered, and to make sure that there is not a lot of overlap or redundancy.

Departmental seminar program

If you are asked to organize a departmental seminar program, chances are that this program has a history. Find out who has organized this program in the past. Such people have considerable experience to share with you. Find out who has previously participated in the program as a speaker. This will give you a good idea of the expectations of your audience and will enable you to avoid being repetitious with speakers or subjects.

Solicit suggestions for potential speakers from others in your department, and try to select a range of different speakers so that everyone will find something interesting in the program. Talk to each visiting speaker and to people who have previously visited your department and ask for suggestions about other speakers who would be of interest. This is a good way to identify younger and less well-known speakers who may have an exciting story to tell.

Organization

As was the case in preparing a talk, the next step is organization. However, "organization" has now expanded to include some additional duties.

Start working on your program as early as possible. The best speakers may have very busy schedules. Start contacting potential speakers immediately. Follow up your telephone calls with something in writing, to remind your speakers that you are really interested in their participation and to confirm the date and time of their presentation.

Make at least one more follow-up call, perhaps two weeks prior to the event. This will serve to remind your speakers of the event. If there are problems at this point, you will have some time to work them out. This is also a good time to inquire about the speaker's audiovisual requirements.

As we suggested previously, talk to people who have done this before. Each one will have some useful suggestions for you. You will hear some cautionary tales about the things which can go wrong, too. Take notes, and if you hear particularly useful ideas please tell *us* about them.

If your program includes both in-house and external speakers, be sure to treat your in-house colleagues just as well as you do the guests. Don't take them for granted or assume that they already know everything they need to know about your program.

Do you have a budget? Do you need to raise funds? Can you offer reimbursement to speakers who must travel? Find out what kind of resources you have available.

When you are inviting your speakers, do so in writing. Each speaker should have a single piece of paper which tells:

- The theme of the program
- When the speaker will be speaking
- The schedule for the day, including when the entire program begins and ends
- How much time the speaker has to speak, and how much time will be available for discussion
- Where the meeting will take place, including an address, directions, and, if necessary, a map
- A telephone number for the speaker to call in case there is difficulty finding the location
- An address, telephone number, fax number, and e-mail address where the speaker can contact you if any questions or problems arise prior to the conference

In a multi-speaker program it's a good idea to let each speaker know who else is participating. If I know that Professor Mueller is talking about his ATPase work and it overlaps with what I am doing, I may then choose to focus on a different aspect of my work rather than repeat material he will be discussing. I may even choose to call him in advance to make sure we aren't duplicating our efforts.

Chairing a program

When you chair a program you *really* have to be prepared to take control. When you were a speaker, part of your job was to make the audience feel comfortable. As the program chairperson your job is to make both the audience and the speakers feel as though everything is under control.

Your actions will set the tone for the whole session. There are several things you should do in advance, and there are responsibilities to be carried out during the program.

In preparation

There are several things to be done in advance of your program. Before the session starts, make sure the room is ready. Arrive early enough to go through the following checklist:

- Is all of the audiovisual equipment working properly? Can everyone see the speaker and the screen? Can speakers be heard clearly throughout the room?
- Do you know where to find spare projector bulbs, or who to contact in case of equipment problems?
- Is there a pointer available?
- Is there adequate seating?
- Are you able to provide a glass of water for each speaker who needs it?
- Are you able to direct speakers and audience to the nearest rest room facilities?

How to introduce a speaker

One of your tasks will be to introduce each speaker, so call each one in advance. Make sure you know the speaker's name (including correct pronunciation), affiliation, and the title of the talk. If you are giving a more elaborate introduction, find out everything you need to know for this purpose ahead of time. When the person doing the introduction has to ask the speaker about his or her education, experience, or title during the introduction, it appears to the audience that the introducer is unprepared. Let your speakers know you are making an introduction so that the speaker will not also be preparing an introduction.

The introduction should be *brief!* Do not use up the speaker's precious time. Just provide the essential information to the audience. Be *certain* to mention the speaker's name and affiliation, as well as the title of the talk. A short summary of the speaker's qualifications (education, work experience, and awards, for example) is also a good idea, but don't be encyclopedic about this – just hit the high points so that people know the speaker is worth listening to. Be sure you do not steal the speaker's thunder by telling too much about the subject of the talk. This is like giving away the surprise ending of a book or movie.

It is particularly pleasing if your introduction tells something about the speaker which helps to personalize or connect the speaker to the audience. This could be a personal anecdote if you know the person well enough. It could be a way in which the speaker's path has crossed yours or your institution's. It could be a common interest outside the subject of the talk. It should present the speaker as an interesting human being with a story to tell, and it should not embarrass anyone.

Running the show

You may wish to provide a few introductory remarks. Be enthusiastic about your program. This is your opportunity to set a positive tone for the whole session. You should also state the theme of the session. For example: "We are really fortunate to have such a distinguished group of speakers this morning. In the past five years photomask design has grown into a 10 billion dollar industry. We will be hearing about the latest results from three of the best labs in the industry." Your introductory remarks are also an appropriate place to publicly acknowledge sponsors of your program or other people who have helped to organize the event. But keep these remarks brief – the invited speakers are the main event.

One of your responsibilities is to control the timing of the session. Start on time. If you wait for all of the stragglers you will never get started. Once you begin, people will rapidly find their places. Let speakers and audience know what the timetable is. You may wish to give your speakers a subtle cue to let them know they have five minutes left. You may need to have a not-so-subtle cue for when the time has expired. Be sure your speakers are aware of the time limits and your signals. What kind of cues? There are numerous possibilities: a timer which beeps, a flashing flashlight, a gentle tap of the gavel; a word from the chairperson; we have even seen a small stuffed animal thrown at speakers who exceed their limit, although this seems a little extreme!

Once you have gotten the speaker to stop speaking you may need to take charge of a question-and-answer or discussion session after the talk. Some speakers are able to manage these sessions on their own, and some may need help. Be prepared to do the following:

- Select questioners.
- Make sure everyone has an opportunity to participate – don't let one questioner monopolize the speaker's time.
- Make sure that each question is repeated so that everyone can hear.
- Draw the discussion session to a close when the time has run out.
- If the speaker has already used up all of the time available you can request that questioners hold their questions until after the session is over and see the speaker on an individual basis.

Often at large national conferences there are people coming and going throughout the session. If necessary, take a moment between speakers to allow people to move in and out of the room. You may wish to point out where empty seats are available to make this process more efficient.

Be certain that each speaker gets applause. If you start applauding, everyone will join in. Don't be tentative – just start clapping.

At the end of the session be prepared to make a few concluding remarks. It is particularly rewarding to the speakers if you briefly mention something you learned from each talk, and this may also serve as a useful summary for the listeners. This is also an appropriate time to express your appreciation to the speakers, the audience, and any sponsors or people who helped to organize the session.

After the show is over

After the program, take a moment to thank each speaker individually. It's a good idea to follow this up with a written note of thanks within a few days. You know by now the effort required to give a good presentation. Your acknowledgment lets people know their efforts were appreciated, and it makes them more likely to be receptive the next time you need their help.

Summary

Organizing a program with several speakers is similar in some ways to organizing a single talk. You may need to establish a key message or theme, you need to analyze the audience, and you need to organize. You also need to devote extra attention to room arrangements and you must introduce your speakers properly. Keep the program on schedule, and afterwards thank those who have participated.

Some key messages from this chapter

- *For a symposium or a group presentation, identify the theme or key message.*
- *Communicate with your speakers to inform them of the arrangements, expectations, time constraints, and facilities available. Find out what their audiovisual requirements will be.*
- *When chairing a program, make certain that all arrangements are in order before the session starts. Take control of the session so that the program runs on time. Give each speaker a positive, but brief, introduction.*
- *After the program is over, be sure to thank the speakers for their efforts.*

Exercise

What is your favorite technical topic? Imagine that you are asked to organize a one-day program on this subject, with a substantial travel budget. What would be the title and theme of your program? Who would you invite to speak? How much time would you allow for each speaker?

Concluding remarks

In the listener's mind, the quality of your presentation reflects on the quality of your work, your organization, your product. If your talk seems pointless or dull, your work, your organization or your product will be assumed pointless and unexciting. Oral presentations are your opportunity to connect immediately with people, quickly build your professional credibility and make sure your messages are impressed on people's minds. This cannot be assured by the use of a written presentation. When you convey life and enthusiasm in a talk by being "you at your best," listeners will be enthusiastic about your message. Your message will come to life, be memorable, and gain your hoped-for results.

In this book we have described the importance of developing a key message. Once you have done this the task of organizing your talk will be greatly simplified, and your ability to be calm and in control of questions will be improved. After you have organized your talk it will be easy to decide what kinds of visual aids best support your message. The key message serves both as a foundation on which your talk is built and as a focal point to keep you on track instead of trying to tell your audience everything you know about your topic. It will keep you from being distracted by an impertinent question. Listeners are more impressed by clarity than by technical detail.

We have devoted several chapters to the mechanics of speaking: using your voice, choosing appropriate words, pausing, making eye contact, and using effective gestures. Remember to focus on one aspect at a time, work on it until you can do it automatically, and then move on to another. If you try to work on everything at once you may feel overwhelmed. You are the most important visual component of the presentation, and each effort you make to put yourself into your presentation and connect more with the audience is a significant step forward. Being a great speaker starts with a sincere desire to communicate and is an ongoing effort to build skill upon skill over time.

Finally, we want to emphasize the value of practice. Take every opportunity to stand up in front of people and talk. You will find that you are less fearful and more successful with every experience. You will gain a skill which you can use for the rest of your life, wherever your career takes you and in your everyday life. An excellent technical professional who can communicate ideas in an oral presentation will be respected as a leader and a valued team member. Share your presentation skill with others and create many worthwhile, professional occasions. We are constantly looking for ways to improve oral technical communication. If you have suggestions, comment, or experience you would like to share, please send them to us (eric.walters@finchcms.edu).

The speaker's bookshelf

There are numerous books on public speaking and the art of oral presentation. Unfortunately, almost all of them are aimed at salespeople or business presentations. We have found the following books to be particularly helpful for technical speaking.

Ailes, R., *You Are the Message: Getting What You Want by Being Who You Are*, Doubleday, New York, 1988.

Anholt, R.R.H., *Dazzle 'em with Style: The Art of Oral Scientific Presentation*, W.H. Freeman, New York, 1994.

Buzan, T. and Buzan, B., *The Mind Map Book*, Dutton, New York, 1993.

Leech, T., *How to Prepare, Stage, and Deliver Winning Presentations*, Amacom, New York, 1982.

Mckerrow, R.E., Gronbeck, B.E., Ehinger, D., and Monroe, A.H., *Principles and Types of Speech Communication*, 14th Edition, Allyn & Bacon, Boston, Mass., 1999.

Peoples, D.A., *Presentations Plus*, John Wiley & Sons, New York, 1988.

Sarnoff, D., *Never Be Nervous Again*, Ivy Books, New York, 1989.

Sindermann, C., *Winning the Games Scientists Play*, Plenum Press, New York, 1982.

Tufte, E.R., *The Visual Display of Quantitative Information*, Graphics Press, Cheshire, Conn., 1983.

Index

action 24
adapting material 103, 111–17;
  adapting written material for oral
  presentation 112–13; change of
  audience 111, 113–15; change of
  length 115–16; checklist 117;
  reason for adapting 111–12
adding to transparencies 42, 43
AIDA 23–4
Ailes, Roger 83
analogies 13, 83–4
Anholt, Robert 23, 36
anticipating questions 8–9, 97
arms 92–3
arranging ideas 26–7
attention 24
attitude 73–4
audience 3–7, 74; adapting material
  for a different audience 111, 113–
  15; consideration for in question
  and answer sessions 99–100;
  expectations 6–7, 35–6, 73;
  finding out about 4–5; non-native
  language audience 86–7; occasion
  for presentation 4; sensitivity to
  10; talking to before presentation
  70; technical knowledge 5–6, 12

backgrounds 50
bar graphs 53, 54
blackboards 46, 58
body language see nonverbal
  communication
body of presentation 19–21

Borden, Richard C. 24–5
borders 50
breathing 81
bullet charts 51–2
Buzan, Tony 28

calmness 105, 108
chairing multi-speaker programs
  121–4; control 123–4; introducing
  speakers 122–3; preparation 122;
  thanking speakers 124
clarity 13–14
close-ended questions 107–8
collecting ideas 26–7
colors 50
comments 99
complete sentences 33
computer projection 47, 58
computer software 49–50
conclusion 14, 21–2, 76
conclusions, significant 11
confidence 82
context 9, 18–19
contrast 50
control 67, 69–77; before
  presentation 69, 70–1; beginning
  presentation 69, 71–3; multi-
  speaker programs 121–2, 123–4;
  throughout presentation 69, 73–6
crises 108–9

D'Angelo, Lihong 86
delivery 67; see also control,
  language, nonverbal

89 71 BR **7906**
      FM
02/03 04-172-00 GBC